Praise for *Staff Educator's Guide to Professional Development*

"Nursing competence is a critical component in ensuring patient safety. In this book, Jeffery, Longo, and Nienaber offer staff educators a road map to successfully fulfill their role in helping nurses develop, maintain, and continuously improve their competence."

–Beth Ulrich, EdD, RN, FACHE, FAAN
Professor, University of Texas Health Science Center at
Houston School of Nursing
Editor, *Nephrology Nursing Journal*

"Staff Educator's Guide to Professional Development *is a fine addition to your nursing professional development library. The highly qualified authors have produced a book written in an informal, conversational style that is easy to comprehend. Especially helpful are the innovative Questions for Reflection/Discussion and Key Takeaways included at the end of each chapter. The reflection questions encourage the nursing professional development specialist to think critically. The Key Takeaways help to highlight important points of information. I think you will enjoy reading this book."*

–Adrianne E. Avillion, DEd, RN
CEO, Strategic Nursing Professional Development

"Staff Educator's Guide to Professional Development: Assessing and Enhancing Nurse Competency *is written in an engaging, conversational manner that makes you feel as though you are in conversation with a trusted mentor helping you improve skills and knowledge in your professional development role. Clinical wisdom is shared, with tables, charts, and practical samples that can be applied to your practice immediately. The chapter on 'putting technology to work' is especially helpful, given that many of us feel challenged to keep up with changing trends and technologies. The handbook has the right balance of theory and practice to ensure the nurse educator is well equipped to employ educational interventions that will ultimately improve patient care."*

–Vicky R. Bowden, DNSc, RN
Vice Provost for Undergraduate Programs and
WASC Accreditation Liaison Officer (ALO)
Azusa Pacific University

"The book does not stop with workforce onboarding and competence validation, but reminds us of the legal and regulatory nature of healthcare—and the reality of lifelong nurse competence with which we have been entrusted. This is a must-read for those of us who will make it our life's work to ensure practicing nurses are competent to care for the health and safety of our public in a high-stakes industry."

–Francine Kingston, DrPH, MSN, RN-BC
Assistant Professor
The University of Texas Health Science Center at Houston
School of Nursing

Staff Educator's Guide to Professional Development

Assessing and Enhancing Nurse Competency

Alvin D. Jeffery, MSN, RN-BC, CCRN-K, FNP-BC
M. Anne Longo, PhD, MBA, RN-BC, NEA-BC
Angela Nienaber, MSN, RN-BC

Sigma Theta Tau International
Honor Society of Nursing®

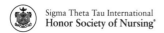

Sigma Theta Tau International
Honor Society of Nursing®

The Honor Society of Nursing, Sigma Theta Tau International (STTI) is a nonprofit organization founded in 1922 whose mission is to support the learning, knowledge, and professional development of nurses committed to making a difference in health worldwide. Members include practicing nurses, instructors, researchers, policymakers, entrepreneurs and others. STTI's 499 chapters are located at 698 institutions of higher education throughout Australia, Botswana, Brazil, Canada, Colombia, Ghana, Hong Kong, Japan, Kenya, Malawi, Mexico, the Netherlands, Pakistan, Portugal, Singapore, South Africa, South Korea, Swaziland, Sweden, Taiwan, Tanzania, United Kingdom, United States and Wales. More information about STTI can be found online at www.nursingsociety.org.

Sigma Theta Tau International
550 West North Street
Indianapolis, IN, USA 46202

To order additional books, buy in bulk, or order for corporate use, contact Nursing Knowledge International at 888.NKI.4YOU (888.654.4968/US and Canada) or +1.317.634.8171 (outside US and Canada).

To request a review copy for course adoption, e-mail solutions@nursingknowledge.org or call 888. NKI.4YOU (888.654.4968/US and Canada) or +1.317.634.8171 (outside US and Canada).

To request author information, or for speaker or other media requests, contact Marketing, Honor Society of Nursing, Sigma Theta Tau International at 888.634.7575 (US and Canada) or +1.317.634.8171 (outside US and Canada).

ISBN: 9781940446264
EPUB ISBN: 9781940446271
PDF ISBN: 9781940446288
MOBI ISBN: 9781940446295

Library of Congress Cataloging-in-Publication Data

Jeffery, Alvin D., 1986- , author.
Staff educator's guide to professional development: assessing and enhancing nurse competency / Alvin D. Jeffery, M. Anne Longo, Angela Nienaber.
  p. ; cm.
Includes bibliographical references.
ISBN 978-1-940446-26-4 (print : alk. paper) -- ISBN 978-1-940446-27-1 (epub)
-- ISBN 978-1-940446-28-8 (pdf) -- ISBN 978-1-940446-29-5 (mobi)
I. Longo, Anne, 1955- , author. II. Nienaber, Angela, 1965- , author. III. Sigma Theta Tau International, issuing body. IV. Title.
[DNLM: 1. Clinical Competence. 2. Education, Nursing, Continuing--standards. 3. Ethics, Nursing. 4. Staff Development--standards. WY 18.5]
  RT51
610.73--dc23
                          2015028248

First Printing, 2015

Publisher: Dustin Sullivan   Principal Book Editor: Carla Hall
Acquisitions Editor: Emily Hatch   Development and Project Editor: Jennifer Lynn
Editorial Coordinator: Paula Jeffers   Copy Editor: Charlotte Kughen
Cover Designer: Michael Tanamachi   Proofreader: Todd Lothery
Interior Design: Katy Bodenmiller   Indexer: Larry D. Sweazy
Illustrations and Page Layout: Amy Hassos

Dedication

To nurses, who understand the importance of education in delivering compassionate and competent care to the world's people. And to the educators who help nurses grow and develop professionally in their ability to provide that care.

Acknowledgments

We would all like to thank our editors—Emily Hatch, Carla Hall, Jennifer Lynn, and Charlotte Kughen—for their guidance, patience, and attention to detail. We also would like to thank Sigma Theta Tau International for this wonderful opportunity.

Alvin would like to thank his partner Jamey, who not only allowed him to write another book but also supported him in the effort.

Anne would like to acknowledge all of the nurses who came before and those who will follow, as they helped to influence our "presence."

Angie would like to thank her family and friends, who have supported her through this endeavor.

About the Authors

Alvin D. Jeffery, MSN, RN-BC, CCRN-K, FNP-BC

Alvin D. Jeffery, co-author of the award-winning *Staff Educator's Guide to Clinical Orientation: Onboarding Solutions for Nurses*, is a full-time PhD student at Vanderbilt University and a predoctoral Quality Scholar Nurse Fellow with the U.S. Department of Veterans Affairs, both in Nashville, Tennessee. He holds part-time positions as an education consultant with Cincinnati Children's Hospital Medical Center in Cincinnati, Ohio, and as an adjunct instructor with several colleges and universities.

Before returning to full-time school, Jeffery's most recent job was working as the unit-based educator in a pediatric intensive care unit at Cincinnati Children's Hospital Medical Center. He is board certified in both Nursing Professional Development (American Nurses Credentialing Center) and Pediatric Critical-Care Nursing (American Association of Critical-Care Nurses), and he has developed and instructed internal review courses for both of these certifications.

Jeffery has facilitated several internal services/continuing education programs in various aspects of nursing professional and staff development, and has served as a preceptor for several new educators in the pediatric intensive care unit. He has collaborated with almost every department in the organization, design, and development of various staff development projects including, but not limited to, competency assessment tools, education record management databases, simulation implementation, and preceptor development.

M. Anne Longo, PhD, MBA, RN-BC, NEA-BC

M. Anne Longo has worked in staff development for 25 years, 9 of them as the senior director for the Center for Professional Excellence/Education at Cincinnati Children's Hospital Medical Center. Longo's other professional roles include business director for two medical divisions, where she managed staff, operations, and grant budgets. She also spent 4 years as a physician liaison for the community. Longo is board certified in American Nurses Credentialing Center's Nursing Professional Development and as an Advanced Executive in Nursing Administration. Her work has been published in journal articles and book chapters, and her PhD dissertation focused on staff perceptions of the healthy work environment. She developed and taught a PhD course on Assessment and Evaluation for Rocky Mountain University of Health Professions. Her innovations in staff development include RNs being able to access free online Nursing Grand Rounds; the development of a live and online course to prepare pediatric RNs for certification, which was recognized in *Training* magazine's 2008 top 125 list; implementation of an online procedure manual; and a 3-year development plan for staff development educators. Longo worked with the Children's Hospitals Solutions for Patient Safety to design education for prevention standards. She is a member of the American Association of Critical-Care Nurses, Society of Pediatric Nurses, and Sigma Theta Tau International Omicron Omicron Chapter, and she has served on several committees.

Angela Nienaber, MSN, RN-BC

Angela Nienaber currently works as an education consultant for the Center for Professional Excellence/Education at Cincinnati Children's Hospital Medical Center. Prior to being in this role, she was a unit-based educator for the Cardiac Step-Down Unit at Cincinnati Children's Hospital Medical Center. Nienaber has also served as adjunct clinical faculty at the Christ College of Nursing and Health Sciences. She has been involved in staff development for more than 20 years in both pediatric and adult care settings, and she has assisted in the development of orientation competency tools as well as preceptor development. Nienaber is certified in Nursing Professional Development through the American Nurses Credentialing Center. She is also an active member of the American Association of Critical-Care Nurses, serving on the local Cincinnati chapter's Board of Directors.

Table of Contents

Introduction

"I never teach my pupils; I only attempt to provide the conditions in which they can learn."

–Albert Einstein

Welcome to the *Staff Educator's Guide to Professional Development*. If you read the book that kick-started this series (*Staff Educator's Guide to Clinical Orientation: Onboarding Solutions for Nurses*), this quote by Einstein might sound familiar. We use this quote once again because it's also the philosophy that supports our goal in writing this book: We aim to provide you with a written guide on how to provide your learners an environment that is most conducive for their professional learning, growth, and development. This book is about how to help professional nurses maintain and grow their competence—and it includes quite a bit of application for other healthcare providers, too—so that these professionals may provide excellent care for the people they serve.

From assessing and evaluating competency to developing creative learning activities to revising large educational programs, this book explores the nuts and bolts of nursing professional development practice (along with some theory) related to promoting competency.

But what's so special about this book, and why shouldn't you purchase a different one to meet your needs? Without trying to sound overly biased, we acknowledge that there are a lot of amazing books and resources out there that move into great depth for many of the topics we discuss (in fact, we reference many of them). What this book brings to the table is a concise overview and holistic approach to all things professional development specialists might need to perform their duties. The intent of this book is to be your one-stop shop, but in the cases where we think you might want to explore certain topics in more depth, we include some of our favorite resources.

We hope this book serves as a foundational reference guide as well as a just-in-time aid to making your competency assessment and educational delivery programs successful. We believe that when leaders promote strong educational programs and clinicians maintain their maximal competency, care delivery is at its finest. We also believe that day-to-day problems and opportunities arise frequently in the healthcare environment, and sometimes you just need to put out the fire. This book can help you thrive in both of these situations. Through frequent examples and ready-to-use worksheets, this book meets you wherever you are in your journey as a professional development specialist.

Speaking of your journey, you don't have to carry the title of educator or professional development specialist to benefit from this book. The intended audience includes the professionals who hold these titles as well as the mid-level managers, charge nurses, and even clinically advanced bedside nurses who are considered the leaders in their practice settings. Our experience tells us that these are the healthcare leaders who do a lot of the work around competency assessment and promoting nursing professional development, yet they frequently lack the formal training that can help them be most successful. This book can't award you a master's degree in nursing education, but it can give you the essential foundations that will help you thrive in your role. Although not the primary audience, academic educators might find the book helpful in teaching nursing education courses, and senior-level administrators might glean new insights on how to turn visions into reality.

Following is an overview of each chapter so that you can jump right to the section you need. You'll find that we have organized the majority of this book according to the ADDIE model. ADDIE stands for Analyze, Design, Develop, Implement, and Evaluate and is an instructional design framework that has been used extensively in the field. This framework might look similar to the nursing process used every moment in the practice setting. We hope this helps make the transition from the practice of clinical nursing to the practice of education more seamless. As we move through each chapter, we dive more fully into the model. And if the ADDIE model doesn't quite click with you, you might consider the ASSURE model (described in the following feature), which is just as applicable to the content we have included.

ASSURE—WHEN THE ADDIE MODEL DOESN'T MEET YOUR NEEDS

Chapter 3, "Designing and Developing Professional Development Activities," offers information on learning theories to consider as frameworks for which instructional design model to use, but in the meantime, in addition to the ADDIE model, the staff educator may choose to use ASSURE (Heinich, Molenda, Russell, & Smaldino, 1996):

A – Analyze learners.

S – State standards and objectives.

S – Select strategies, technology, media, and materials.

U – Use technology, media, and materials.

R – Require learner participation.

E – Evaluate and revise.

Each staff educator must develop his or her own standards for the practice of education. Having standards for how you perform each of the components of the ADDIE model (or ASSURE) helps you work with staff members to ensure they continue to be lifelong learners who meet the expectations of patients and managers.

We hope you find time someday to read this entire book, but in case you have a fire that needs extinguished right now, here's a preview of where to look:

Chapter 1—"Overview of Professional Development: The Practice of Education": We start with defining what we mean by "professional development" and the various topics it encompasses. In this chapter, we answer questions such as:

- What are professional development, competency, continuing education (CE), and so on?

- Why are educational programs important to patients, staff members, and the organization?

- Who are the important stakeholders necessary for successful professional development?

We then introduce the instructional design model that serves as the outline for the rest of the book. The ADDIE model (Analyze, Design, Develop, Implement, and Evaluate) is a timeless framework used by professional development specialists in healthcare and non-healthcare settings. You're probably already using it (even if you don't realize it).

Chapter 2—"Analyzing the Need for Professional Development Activities": We jump right in to the ADDIE model with Chapter 2, where we look at the *A*—Analysis. In this chapter, we explore how to gather data and information about the need for a professional development activity (as opposed to what might be more of an organizational or management activity). There are many ways to determine what an organization or its employees need, and we attempted to cover almost all of them. In addition to identifying these needs, which can vary over time, we begin to discuss some of the regulatory requirements that exist and how you incorporate these mandates into your needs assessment. We finish the chapter by teaching you how to prepare your findings and present them to others.

Chapter 3—"Designing and Developing Professional Development Activities": Whereas Chapter 2 focuses on establishing *what* the need is, this chapter helps you focus on *how* you'll meet the need. We lay a bit of groundwork on some well-respected learning theories and models that are essential for professional development specialists, and then we use that background to Design and Develop (the next two steps in the ADDIE model) learning activities and educational programs that work for your organization. Each organization is different, comprising unique resources and limitations, so our approach at this point is adaptable to most any setting. That changes in the next chapter.

Chapter 4—"Implementing Professional Development Activities": If Chapter 3 feels a little too generic, you might be the type of learner who wants lots of practical ideas and tools. This chapter is where the rubber meets the road, and we explore the Who, What, When, Where, and Why of learning activities in this fourth step of the ADDIE model— Implement. We look at questions such as:

- Who should (and shouldn't) be the participants of a learning activity?

- What tools and resources are needed for a successful activity, and what is the budget?

- When is the best time to perform a learning activity?

- Where is the environment/location that is most conducive to learning?

- Why is this all being done, and do the learners understand this reason, too?

This chapter could easily be the most important one you read if you're looking for the nuts and bolts of putting a learning activity together. The previous chapters started with a broad scope and narrowed to a specific activity, but this chapter contains many ideas and practical tips for making the learning activity a success.

Chapter 5—"Evaluating an Individual's Growth": After you implement your learning activity or educational program, you always want to know how well it went by doing an Evaluation (the final stage in the ADDIE model). We cover this topic in two chapters because we tend to separately evaluate individual learners and the activity or program. In this chapter, we dive into the definitions of competency and the various ways to measure it. We also look at related concepts, such as critical thinking and interpersonal communication. We then spend time exploring what to do when it looks like competency might not be present.

Chapter 6—"Evaluating an Educational Program's Performance": In addition to how well individual learners perform following a learning activity, we want to step back and examine the big picture of the small learning activity or large educational program we have designed, developed, and implemented. We answer questions like:

- Was offering this learning activity/educational program beneficial to patients, clinicians, and/or the organization?
- Should we offer this activity/program again in the future? If so, how might we offer it differently next time?
- Is the benefit of offering this activity/program worth its costs?

Chapter 7—"Ethical and Legal Considerations": Whew! Moving through the entire ADDIE model took up most of the book! However, we would be remiss if we didn't cover a few other odds and ends that surface from time to time. In this chapter, we look at issues such as board-recognized continuing education (CE) activities: when to offer them, how to apply for them, and what special rules and regulations separate them from non-CE activities. We also bring up licensure and certification: how to help staff members meet requirements for licensure renewal, why it's important to promote certification, and how to help learners prepare for certification exams. We finish the chapter by covering documentation: how and where to keep records of learning activities, what length of time to keep the records, and how to maintain confidentiality.

Chapter 8—"Putting Technology to Work for You": Closely related to both the Implementation chapter (Chapter 4) as well as the ethics and legality chapter (Chapter 7), we devote a chapter to the use of technology. We provide several options (many of which are free) for keeping yourself organized and enhancing learning activities. To keep you organized, we look at how to store electronic records locally as well as the role of premade learning management systems. When it comes to the learners, as long as you have a computer and the Internet, there are endless opportunities for beefing up your learning activities to get participants more engaged. Finally, we look at the role professional development specialists commonly play with respect to technology used for patient care (for example, training staff members on new or updated equipment).

We hope the insight and experiences we share within these pages enrich your practice and move you to enjoy the practice of nursing professional development as much as we do. Finally, as leaders in healthcare, may we not forget the timeless words spoken by Florence Nightingale:

> *"Let whoever is in charge keep this simple question in her head (not, how can I always do this right thing myself, but) how can I provide for this right thing to be always done?"*

> *–Florence Nightingale*

Whether you're new to leading orientation efforts or a seasoned nursing staff development specialist, we think you will find this book a great addition to your personal library. Once you've finished reading it, we hope you'll have new perspectives, found a greater insight, or at least gained a few nuggets of how to do some things better. Regardless of what you discover along the way, we hope you enjoy the journey through these pages as much as we enjoy sharing them with you!

References

Heinich, R., Molenda, M., Russell, J. D., & Smaldino, S. E. (1996). *Instructional media and technologies for learning* (5th ed.). Columbus, OH: Merrill.

Overview of Professional Development: The Practice of Education

Introduction

Historically, the work of the nursing professional development specialist (or a staff educator) focused on orientation of newly hired registered nurses (RNs), inservicing of new products and equipment, continuing education (CE) activities, and student services. Then came the implementation of shared governance, Magnet programs, Pathway to Excellence journeys, and a host of other current trends in the healthcare and nursing environment. Now we commonly see the role of staff educators expanding to serve as shared governance facilitators, which makes sense given that education is the backbone of how the individual nurse learner practices. (A *shared governance facilitator* provides guidance to staff involved in representing their professional roles in decisions regarding their practice.) Staff educators are also found championing change projects or improvement initiatives. This chapter looks at the role of today's professional development specialist as well as the development goals and activities associated with this role.

The Nursing Professional Development Specialist

The role of the staff educator, as the nursing professional development specialist was known early on, expanded beginning in the late 1970s and early '80s as hospital-based schools of nursing began to close, and newly hired RNs were graduates of all types of nursing programs. Although the role evolved for some time (and still does), the American Nurses Association and National Nursing Staff Development Organization's (now known as the Association for Nursing Professional Development) *Nursing Professional Development: Scope and Standards of Practice* (2010) helped to update the key roles by discussing factors such as evidence-based practice (EBP), globalization, technology, and practice environments. The scope and standards manual provides a well-organized systems model with which staff educators should become familiar. The scope and standards are the framework for the nursing professional development specialist's own professional development journey to being an expert in the field as he or she guides the practice of education. In addition, the manual includes measurement criteria to assist educators in ensuring the competency of their own work. The measurement criteria are generic enough to allow individuals to outline how to meet the criteria within their own facility and can be used as a means of self-assessment. Given the evolving role of the professional development specialist, the scope, standards, and measurement criteria can help nurses working in this educator role to consider their own professional development (which could also include the goal of becoming certified through the American Nurses Credentialing Center, or ANCC).

Briefly, the standards by which staff educators could evaluate themselves and their work are found in Table 1.1.

TABLE 1.1 *STANDARDS OF PRACTICE FOR NURSING PROFESSIONAL DEVELOPMENT SPECIALISTS*

PRACTICE

Standard 1: Assessment

Standard 2: Identification of Issues and Trends

Standard 3: Outcomes Identification

Standard 4: Planning

Standard 5: Implementation

   Standard 5A: Coordination

   Standard 5B: Learning and Practice Environment

   Standard 5C: Consultation

Standard 6: Evaluation

PROFESSIONAL PERFORMANCE

Standard 7: Quality of Nursing Professional Development Practice

Standard 8: Education

Standard 9: Professional Practice Evaluation

Standard 10: Collegiality

Standard 11: Collaboration

Standard 12: Ethics

Standard 13: Advocacy

Standard 14: Research

Standard 15: Resource Utilization

Standard 16: Leadership

Source: ANA (2010).

Although it's not required that you have the title of "staff educator" or "professional development specialist," the preceding ANA standards and concepts give you an idea of the functional role of this professional. These leaders do more than direct the actions of a group; they assist others in empowering and achieving outcomes and goals. Professional development specialists are responsible for assisting staff members in maintaining competencies, advancing and growing in their professional practice, assisting in the achievement of career goals, and promoting lifelong learning. Not only are staff educators responsible for planning and implementing learning activities, but they also act as change agents, researchers, and mentors/coaches.

Depending on the unique needs of your organization, these professionals might be called "manager," "charge nurse," or even "clinical nurse specialist." All these titles imply additional responsibilities, but they could easily include some of the activities listed in Table 1.1. Throughout this book, we use the titles "professional development specialist" and "staff educator"—or just "educator"—interchangeably, but we always use these titles to designate the functional role of this professional rather than a specific job position.

The Goal of Nursing Professional Development

Now that you have a vague idea of *who* the staff educator is, this chapter begins with an introductory discussion of how to frame the educators' tasks (for example, orientation, inservicing, and CE) in light of their influence on the caregiver nurse, as well as other members of the interprofessional team, to meet the Triple Aim Initiative of the Institute for Healthcare Improvement (IHI, 2015):

- Improving the patient experience of care (including quality and satisfaction)
- Improving the health of populations
- Reducing the per capita cost of healthcare

Perhaps this description seems like a tall order for the staff educator, but unless you understand how the practice of education influences the practice of nursing, the health of patients will not improve, and the face of healthcare in the United States will not change. In other words, it is an educated nurse acting as the coordinator of patient care and patient advocate who guides patients and their families to better health. And it is the professional development specialist, working in conjunction with nurse leaders, who provides the direct care RN and others with the healthy work environment where lifelong learning can occur.

It truly is up to the 3.1 million U.S. nurses to implement the recommendations in the 2010 Institute of Medicine (IOM) report "The Future of Nursing: Leading Change, Advancing Health." From a professional development specialist role, the key messages are:

- Nursing practice should be based upon the level of education and training.

- Nurses are lifelong learners and should achieve higher levels of education and training through seamless academic progression.

- Nurses should be active in redesigning healthcare with physicians and other health professionals through shared mental models and decision-making.

- Nurses are provided with appropriate data via improved collection and information infrastructure in order to make effective workforce planning and policy-making decisions.

All nurses should be familiar with the most current data-based evidence (whether from research, quality improvement, administrative, or regulatory findings), both about their daily practice and about their changing profession as a whole. The staff educator works with the learners to become knowledgeable about the types and levels of evidence available. Has your facility worked to identify an EBP model to follow? Consider initiating CE activities with a PICO or PICOT (Population, Intervention, Comparison, Outcome, and Time) question, which is a simple way of keeping the need for searching for evidence at the forefront of nurses' learning activities.

As a staff educator, are you comfortable speaking to the summaries of the IHI and IOM reports? Are you familiar with what actions your facility has taken to date? Have you considered how to support these goals within the educator's informal leadership role? To accomplish these large feats, the educator needs to be equipped with knowledge about the following:

- The state's nurse practice act

- The ANA Code of Ethics

- Learning theories and nursing theories

- Competencies

- Nursing philosophy

- Aspects of implementation science

- Instructional design models such as ADDIE

- Regulatory requirements

- Data expectations and repositories

- Current evidence

- The environment for the learner

- The patient population being cared for

- The effect of the education on the learner and the patients

- The cost of the education, including return on investment (ROI)

Acquiring this knowledge might initially seem like a difficult task, but after becoming familiar with the resources and guidance we outline in this book, you'll be much more comfortable with these concepts.

In essence, the goal of the professional development specialist working in any practice setting is to serve as the "knowledge broker" between the learner and the intended education. In this millennium, serving as the knowledge broker means being able to provide the learner with guidance to *integrate* the knowledge, skill, and behaviors to improve nursing practice.

To reinforce the importance of this goal, take a moment to copy the following sentence and post it somewhere you can read it every day:

The goals of the expert educator are to demonstrate both the value of education (cost/benefit) and the transfer of learning to behavior (best practice)!

Source: Adapted from Kirkpatrick & Kirkpatrick (2005).

AN EXAMPLE OF PRACTICE INTEGRATION

As an example of practice integration, consider when and how the professional development specialist would use the ANA Provisions of the Code of Ethics with Interpretive Statements as part of orientation for new graduates.

The Code of Ethics is not new, yet how many orientations, inservices, or CE activities integrate the statements that are appropriate for the content?

Posting the Code of Ethics on each patient care area or clinic as a reminder might be helpful, but demonstrating how to implement and evaluate the interpretive statements is what makes a difference to the caregiving nurse. To facilitate a learner's transition from a state of simply knowing that ethical standards exist to the point of consistently and effectively applying them to every patient situation—that's the goal of the staff educator's work.

To learn more about how the ANA Code of Ethics can be used as one of the frameworks for orientation, see the feature titled "Translating How the ANA Code of Ethics Is Part of Orientation's Framework," in Chapter 7, "Ethical and Legal Considerations."

- *Review the essentials of the facility's safety program every day by asking speakers to include in presentations, simulations, and online modules the specific safety aspects related to their subject. For example, preventing pressure ulcers can be incorporated into presentations related to nutrition, and inspecting the skin can occur during the performance of any procedure.*

- *Discuss how to communicate potential concerns to other health team members such as medical assistants, patient care assistants, physical therapists, and respiratory therapists. Document concerns where other health care members can review or note during change of shift report. Newly hired nurses must learn from the outset the importance of being the coordinator of care and what that means for keeping patient safety at the forefront of daily practice.*

- *Discuss patient safety as part of patient education. Incorporate return demonstration (teach-back) into daily practice. It is still the expectation that discharge planning begins upon admission for inpatients at every office/urgent care/emergency department visit because, from a nursing perspective, planning for discharge is the predominant way to prevent readmissions. Readmissions, as you may already know, is an expectation of the federal government. Again, the nurse learner is improving patient outcomes/experience and decreasing cost to patients and facilities (IHI Triple Aim).*

- *Educate the preceptors on a standardized way to coach new orientees and the responsibility for assessing the progress of orientees in an ethical manner.*

- *Weave the importance of the "Professional Role Competence" ANA Position Statement, reaffirmed November 12, 2014, into orientation.*

While a great deal of time is spent in the learner's acquisition of skill competency, it is the nurse learner's overall behavior that becomes the nurse. It is how the art of nursing care becomes the practice of nursing.

One Challenge of Nursing Professional Development

Today's workforce is a lively mix of generations—five generations of people working side by side for the first time. This mix means you are more likely than ever before to be leading, coaching, and teaching people who are nothing like you at all.

So how do you find common ground? One starting point is to gain an understanding of these generational cohorts. Each generation has its own shared history, common biases, and core beliefs. And different generations care about different approaches to the same problem. For example, is it the case that the technology you were exposed to in your generation might have some effect on the way you learn throughout your life? Ultimately, you need to respect and understand what drives these different generations, what is most important to them, and how they like to learn, and you need to know how to interact with them. Table 1.2 provides brief descriptions of the commonly encountered generational differences.

TABLE 1.2 *OVERVIEW OF THE FIVE GENERATIONS IN THE CURRENT WORKFORCE**

VETERAN GENERATION (BORN BEFORE 1945)

Comprises smallest generation in the workforce

Is driven by ideals of duty and service

Measures work ethic on timeliness, productivity, and not drawing attention to oneself

Values quality over speed and efficiency; does not require fancy options and customization

Is also known as traditionalist, silent generation, and mature

Is influenced by the military and came of age during the Great Depression

Experienced World War II, Pearl Harbor, and Hiroshima

BOOMER GENERATION (BORN 1945–1964)

Comprises one of the largest generations in history and dominates the workforce

Evaluates themselves and others based on work ethic

Have mixed opinions on technology and believe it causes about as many problems as it solves

Are considered the most influential people today who often run local, state, and national governments and are the bosses, supervisors, managers, and CEOs in most companies

Believe in, champion, and evaluate themselves and others based on their work ethic, which is measured in hours spent on the job (leading to the term "workaholic")

Values face time over productivity

GENERATION X (BORN 1965–1982)

Grew up in the "me generation"

Have been taught to question authority

Dismiss the boomers' work-'til-you-drop ethic

Loyal to people rather than organizations

Raised in a world where national institutions seemed to fall like dominoes as church scandals, impeachments, and divorce were almost a regular occurrence

Seek open communication regardless of position, title, or tenure

Have a prove-it-to-me attitude

Are more skeptical and cynical than earlier generations and have no shared heroes

Believe productivity on the job matters more than time on the job

Want to control the decision and the plan, selecting options that make sense to the way they live and work rather than what someone has predetermined for them

Are more interested in quality of life than success at work

Embrace technology and use it in most aspects of their lives to help them produce more work in less time, which can lead to an appropriate work–life balance

continues

TABLE 1.2 *(CONTINUED)*

Are the first generation to have home computers and access to computers in the classroom

Are multitaskers

Don't use TV as a source of entertainment and information

MILLENNIAL GENERATION (BORN 1980–2000)

Is also known as NET Gen, GEN Y, or Generation Why

Raised with terrorist attacks

Is the most overscheduled generation in U.S. history

Likes immediate feedback

Believes information can be acquired very quickly

Have been coddled since birth, have been protected by their parents, and are used to getting a great deal of positive (and immediate) feedback

Seeks ways to shed stress in life

Strive to align themselves with individuals who will help them achieve their goals and are not in awe of authority figures

Seeks open communication

Is better equipped to get along in the diverse, global world than any previous generation

Is a technology-savvy group that has never known a world without cell phones, laptops, or remote controls and can teach others how to use technology

Relies on the Internet rather than TV for entertainment

Reads less than other generations

Craves challenges

GENERATION Z (2000–PRESENT)

Two billion people; most connected, educated, sophisticated generation ever

Is tech-savvy; true digital natives

Have little concern for privacy; no problem sharing the most intimate details with strangers

Able to multitask, which might lead to lack of ability to focus and analyze lengthy information

Thrives on instant gratification; requires short bursts of information to be understood

Includes early adopters, brand influencers, social media drivers, and pop culture leaders

Sources: Mueller (2015), McCrindle (2015), and Shah (2011).

In addition to identifying the generation of the learner, understanding the student's preferred method of learning, and determining the most appropriate educational method for the learner, the professional development specialist needs to bear in mind the following general principles associated with adult learning theory (Patterson, Grenny, Maxfield, McMillan, & Switzler, 2008):

- People choose their behaviors based on what they think will happen to them as a result.

- The factors influencing whether people choose to enact a vital behavior are based on two essential expectations: Is it worth it? Can I do it?

- The great persuader is personal experience.

Although the preceding principles from Patterson's book *Influencer* are based in adult learning theory, those who are working as professional nurse educators can apply them to better guide the learner from novice to expert caregiver. These principles are the reasons we choose different learning modalities depending upon the desired outcomes—for example, simulation of skills, the use of the Socratic method by preceptors, and even the use of observation to ensure learners are applying best practice.

A Google search provides more than 250 infographics on characteristics of the modern learner. Tauber and Johnson (2014) created an infographic called "Meet the Modern Learner" for Bersin by Deloitte. The overarching takeaway from the infographic is that 1% of the workweek is all the typical worker can devote to education. Thus the educator should consider the infographic's three themes— overwhelmed, distracted, and impatient (Tauber & Johnson [2014])— when deciding on approaches to use for specific topics (see Table 1.3).

TABLE 1.3   *CHOOSING EDUCATIONAL APPROACHES THAT MATCH THE THEMES OF TODAY'S LEARNERS*

THEME	APPROACH
Overwhelmed	Regardless of the educational format chosen, integration of new content into existing work is critical to successful application of the new content. If learners perceive the change is not valued because it's not reinforced, it is normal for them to revert to what they initially learned. So if you need to educate learners on a policy change, for example, you should review that policy change at shift change, documentation, patient assessment, and so on to underscore its value.
Distracted	One huge problem in all areas of nursing is competing priorities (beginning with the phone!). Because communication is critical to patient care, always considering how, where, when, why, and to whom education is delivered is essential. For example, if the content requires learners to be away from the work environment, you should set a timeframe for the application of the content. The old adage "use it or lose it" is part of the life of those working in healthcare. (It's why annual competencies are so popular.)
Impatient	Learners in all walks of life want to believe they know what's going on and are contributing to patient, unit, and facility goals. Their impatience is threefold: personal (sick kid, angry spouse, rent due), patient (lots of tasks/caring to provide), and colleague (boss expectations, delegation to support staff issues, tasks left from the previous shift). Educators can use impatience to reinforce safety, communication, and teamwork aspects into all learning activities.

You may identify that these and other themes are affecting learners in your own work environment. Consider also which approaches are working for your learners. How do you know what is working? Check the data: Did incident reports decrease after a learning activity? What does the electronic medical record (EMR) show? When you perform pre/post evaluation of how education is being applied by learners, you are demonstrating that learners value the education (because they applied it) as well as demonstrating your own value as an educator.

Nursing Professional Development Activities

As we continue to define (and refine) what nursing professional development entails, it can be helpful to consider several of the activities that typically fall under its purview. These activities include (but are definitely not limited to) the following:

- Orientation

- Patient education and cultural/diversity awareness

- Inservicing

- Ensuring the value of education

- Quality improvement, evidence-based practice, and research

- Continuing education

- Student services

We introduce you to these activities here and give you some examples and additional information throughout the book.

As we discuss the staff educator's role in various educational activities, we refer to a wide range of activities that are meant to enhance the practice of nurses who have finished their prelicensure, academic work. In other words, we are educating licensed nurses (or in some states a graduate nurse who is about to take the nursing licensure exam). Most of the literature refers to "nurse educators" as those in an academic setting, and the role of a "staff educator" (or "nursing professional development specialist") is quite different from that of a faculty member. The staff educator's role involves building upon academic baseline knowledge and skills in what the ANA refers to as *continuing education (CE)*. We like this term but think it can easily be interpreted as "accredited" CE, which implies those activities necessary for licensure renewal. We want to be more broad than that to also include those activities that might be necessary for other regulatory bodies (for example, the Centers for Medicare and Medicaid Services), organizational needs (for example, changes in policies or equipment), or for an individual's professional growth (for example, certification or advancing on the clinical ladder). See Figure 1.1.

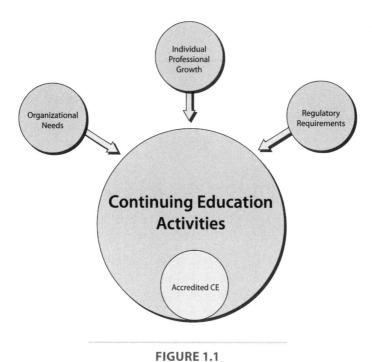

FIGURE 1.1

Continuing education (CE) activities may or may not be accredited.

Orientation

On a simple level, orientation of the newly hired nurse may mean providing resources to new employees that ensure the facility's policies and procedures are implemented correctly. From regulatory requirements (such as how to administer blood or how to apply restraints appropriately) to the who's who of leadership and other disciplines (for example, social services, nutrition, or respiratory therapy), staff educators are intimately involved in an organization's orientation activities.

It is one thing for staff educators to organize the materials, speakers, and so on to ensure orientation activities go off without a hitch. Yet educators who want to socialize the newly hired employee into both the caring profession of nursing and the culture of the institution (known as *onboarding*) should consider incorporating the forthcoming concepts as a means of helping the new nurse make the transition from the academic environment to the practice setting. For educators, this process means using the ADDIE model (Analyze, Design, Develop, Implement, and Evaluate), described in Chapter 2, "Analyzing the Need for Professional Development Activities," to design the orientation activities and communicate the content and expectations to nurse leaders, preceptors, and the newly hired employees.

Staff educators should begin orientation by reviewing the Quality and Safety Education for Nurses competencies (QSEN, 2014) that are based upon the Institute of Medicine competencies for healthcare professionals (IOM, 2003). Funded by the Robert Wood Johnson Foundation, the QSEN Institute is housed in the Frances Payne Bolton School of Nursing at Case Western Reserve University. Academia has defined prelicensure and graduate quality and safety competencies for nursing as including:

- Patient-centered care
- Teamwork and collaboration
- Evidence-based practice
- Quality improvement
- Safety
- Informatics

The following list of core competencies (Interprofessional Education Collaborative Expert Panel, 2011) is comprised of professional roles that include nursing, medicine, dentistry, pharmacy, and even public health. Note, then, the need for educators to include at minimum these competencies in developing staff:

- Provide patient-centered care.
- Use informatics.
- Employ evidence-based practice.
- Apply quality improvement.

The professional development specialist working in a practice setting who is knowledgeable regarding what learners have already learned about the QSEN and interprofessional competencies can tailor the orientation effort to the individual learner. Here, the staff educator acts as the knowledge broker between the learners' academic work and their new practice setting via the orientation program. The staff educator can even perform some of this work before the new employee is hired (and think of some of the cost-saving effects this might have, including increased employee satisfaction and retention). For example, consider using the following activities prior to hire:

- Work closely with human resources to determine whether the applicants can perform an individual learning assessment. Examples include the simple, free, online VARK (Visual, Aural, Read/write, Kinesthetic) test or a simulation that includes knowledge and procedural skills.

- Perform a knowledge assessment of the applicant's QSEN and/or interprofessional competencies.

- Deliver a personality test or values assessment to determine whether applicants will support the changing culture of the work setting.

In other words, the staff educator should *standardize, standardize,* and *standardize* again the responsibilities and expectations of the orientation program. By doing so, the educator ensures that those aspects of nursing requiring consistency—every patient, every time—are never wavered from. The importance of standardization is it allows the nurse learner to then think about the needs of the individual patient. The patient receives care based upon current evidence, and regulatory requirements are met.

Patient Education and Cultural/ Diversity Awareness

At the forefront of the practice of education is the need for the professional development specialist to consider patient education as the focus for "care along the continuum." Consider patient education to be a demonstration of how the profession of nursing meets the patient's expectation of competency regardless of the type of nursing being practiced. Patient education also assists nursing to meet the portion of the IHI's Triple Aim related to population health. Patient education needs to be included in all programs developed by the staff educator, whether it's orientation, an inservice, or a CE activity. What does the patient and family need to learn, when do they need to learn it, and how should it be taught?

Patient and family education begins at the time of admission and should be reinforced on every shift. "Even night shift?" you ask. Consider, for example, if the patient awakens due to the taking of vital signs. Nurses could offer a quiet reminder of *why* that particular patient's vital signs are important to the progression of his or her recovery (that is, has the patient had a fever, redness at the operation site post-operatively that might be a sign of a surgical site infection, and so on?). Educating with a quiet touch and whisper of what is taking place might allow the patient to remain sleepy during the process. Not only mimicking these behaviors (if the staff educator performs clinical work) but also helping nurses understand their role as patient educators are within the professional development specialist's scope of practice.

HELPFUL RESOURCES

Are you feeling overwhelmed yet? If so, know that there are plenty of resources out there to help you, especially with regard to regulatory standards and national expectations. For example, The Joint Commission (www.jointcommission.org), the Centers for Medicare and Medicaid Services (www.cms.gov), the Agency for Healthcare Research & Quality (www.ahrq.gov), the National Quality Forum (www.qualityforum.org), and the Healthcare Education Association (www.hcea-info.org) have free resources on their websites. There is no need to start from scratch. (Just remember to give credit as you tweak the content to meet your patient population's goals.)

ADVICE FOR THE NEW PROFESSIONAL DEVELOPMENT SPECIALIST

As a novice educator, the scope of the practice of education is overwhelming. Most likely, you have been considered an expert in the care of a specific patient population or recently obtained your master's degree. Going from being an expert to a novice might have made you ask, "What was I thinking?" Please know that the same skills you developed that created the expert in one area of practice can be translated to the practice of education. Skills such as time management, relationship building, knowledge of your facility, and even experience with precepting are all necessary for using ADDIE as the instructional design model for the practice of education. Map out your own pathway to becoming an expert professional development educator by using the ANA Nursing Professional Development: Scope and Standards of Practice written for this role to outline your journey to expert educator. It is the educator's passion and believing the nurse learner desires to provide best practice that will help you every day.

Inservicing

Today's professional development specialist is a leader, as are all RNs, regardless of role or practice setting. The major means of leading in the educator role, however, is through influence; translating knowledge, skills, and attitudes (KSAs) into behaviors; and integrating professional, regulatory, and organizational expectations. Inservicing is one of the primary means by which the nurse learner remains up to date with the KSAs necessary to apply EBP to reach desired patient outcomes.

Inservices are activities designed to increase the nurse learner's competence in the professional nurse role at a specific facility. Inservice topics can cover new or updated policies and procedures, or they can be a review of content related to policies and procedures, equipment, regulatory requirements, performance improvement work, patient and employee safety initiatives, population health, unit goals, facility goals, and so on. Almost any KSA that the nurse learner needs in order to provide excellent care on every shift can be partially (if not completely) acquired through an inservice. Now, we're not necessarily talking about inservices in the boring, non-engaging, one-hour lecture sense; instead we mean a unique learning activity that can take on a variety of presentation styles. As a simple example, would you consider including aspects of professional boundaries, emergency preparedness, or your state's Nurse Practice Act for the inservice whose focus happens to be "caring for the patient with a mental health issue"? The content of inservices need not be constrained to a single topic, but it should be possible for the learner to immediately apply it in the care setting.

Inservices are also a wonderful opportunity for the staff educator to include the caring aspects of the art and science of nursing. What is the nursing philosophy of your organization? What are the values of the organization? One way is to always include an aspect of how to communicate with the patient and family, and with each other. Because the literature notes the five generations communicate in different ways, perhaps returning to a simple touch of the patient's hand upon entering or leaving the room, regardless of the reason for entering the room, would communicate caring. And while texting might be the future of checking in with the healthcare professional, it has nothing on a smile or kind word to one who is not feeling well and is expected to make important decisions as a partner in the patient's care.

Ensuring the Value of Education

Another major goal of the nursing professional development specialist is to demonstrate the value of education. In addition to the intrinsic value of professional development, staff educators should examine budgeting (specifically, evaluating a return on investment) for all types of programs. Staff educators can set up working budgets for 1-hour, 4-hour, and even all-day programs. Including guesstimates for the amount of time the staff educator spent planning, implementing, and evaluating as well as the amount of time learners spend in class along with materials, refreshments, and so on will all comprise the budget for a learning activity.

There are many user-friendly budget templates you can find online with a simple search. You can easily send these budget documents, along with the impact of the activities, as monthly or quarterly reports to the organization's leaders to help them understand the impact of the staff educator's role both on the nurse learner and the cost to the facility. (Chapter 6, "Evaluating an Educational Program's Performance," goes into more detail on methods for demonstrating the value of learning activities and educational programs.)

Quality Improvement, Evidence-Based Practice, and Research in the Practice of Education

In reading the chapter to this point, you might have started to recognize that the staff educator's role in performance and quality improvement and EBP should be automatic and threaded throughout all aspects of teaching. These are areas of opportunity for academicians and professional development specialists to standardize approaches for implementing quality improvement and the use of evidence. Standardized approaches assist new graduate nurses in transitioning from school to practice. There are many online resources to guide the educator in learning how to implement quality improvement and EBP. Particularly helpful is the IHI's website at www.ihi.org.

Research in the practice of education as performed in work settings is lacking in the nursing literature. The staff educator should consider this as a goal for being the professional development *expert*. You should reach out to local nurse researchers (if you are located in an academic setting) to look for opportunities for working together. For others, reading literature in the areas of business and education (outside of nursing) can provide different aspects of what you and others in the nursing profession might choose to adopt.

Continuing Education

Continuing education (CE) activities, by definition, are planned and build upon the professional nurse learner's focus, whether it be education, practice, research, administration, or some other field. To help stay organized, the staff educator who designs CE activities should develop an annual chart with the following attributes:

- Requirements of one's state practice act. (As of 2013, 13 states did not require some form of CE to renew the RN license compared to other states that require annual information on human immunodeficiency virus, child abuse, and so on.)

- Requirements of those certified in the various specialties working at your facility.

- Requirements for those desiring to advance via the facility's clinical advancement program (if you have one).

- List of the facility's growth areas. For example, will you be caring for additional patient populations or joining a healthcare system and needing to combine cultures?

- Knowledge of planned changes to various roles that affect the nurse learner. Similarly, when should CE offerings include other disciplines and the content be based in the interprofessional competencies?

Creating such a chart allows the educator to map out programs a year in advance and potentially collaborate with other facilities to offer well-designed, meaningful education to the nurse learner. With the understanding that professional nurses need to embrace lifelong learning as a responsibility for which the individual is accountable, the educator also has the opportunity to use CE activities to generate long-term educational plans as a means of assisting nurse learners to become experts in their area of focus.

Benner's Novice-to-Expert Model (1984) advises that it takes 5 years to become an expert in a specific area (for example, adult medical-surgical, pediatric oncology, or outpatient psychiatry). The educator's focus has predominantly been on initial orientation and keeping staff up to date via inservices. Developing 3- to 5-year plans for nurse learners working in practice settings, the field of education, administration, and research sets the tone for showing learners how they are advancing the profession as well as themselves.

For example, RNs who are board certified in leadership are required to have a specific number of CE contact hours specific to leadership. The American Organization of Nurse Executives (AONE), the ANA Leadership Institute, the American Association of Critical-Care Nurses (AACN), and many other organizations offer leadership competencies for various levels of "line" leaders (as well as to those interested in becoming operational leaders). The staff educator needs to be aware of the requirements and work with the leadership of the facility to determine which competencies to focus on based upon the facility's goals. For example, how does leadership work to support/engage in the patient and employee safety programs?

To illustrate this point, most nursing leadership organizations include a competency on the area of communication. From the literature, the staff educator knows that communication is a major cause of errors (check out The Joint Commission Sentinel Alert 30 and 39, which provide specific examples). Depending upon the work setting of the staff educator, a CE activity for leaders can focus on how to implement standardized communication with staff and patients specific to the care of the facility's patient populations.

> **NOTE**
>
> *A national CE conference was held in the United States for the first time in 1969. The group that chose to continue a conference focused on CE is called PNEG (Professional Nurse Educators Group). The conference is a nice mix of the best of academia and practice, so you might consider subscribing to PNEG on LinkedIn.*

Student Services

Almost all areas of nursing practice provide learning opportunities for students, and in many work settings, it is the staff educator who acts as the liaison between the school of nursing faculty and the practice setting. Depending upon the program level of the student, the nursing professional development specialist must be knowledgeable of the National League for Nursing's report "Outcomes and Competencies for Graduates of Practical/Vocational, Diploma, Associate Degree, Baccalaureate, Master's, Practice Doctorate, and Research Doctorate Programs in Nursing" (NLN, 2010). Together with the QSEN competencies, the educator can work toward assisting the practicing RNs with understanding the current academic expectations of the various levels of students.

As nurse practice leaders work with nurse academic leaders to implement the Robert Wood Johnson Foundation and AARP Future of Nursing initiative to implement and evaluate the 2010 IOM report's recommendations, it is the staff educators who must remain aware and knowledgeable of the program's status within their own state. Educators working in practice settings need to prepare for these changes and how an opportunity to work with school faculty might standardize aspects of nursing care related to specific patient populations.

Staff educators must expand their own practice of education by understanding the competencies of other healthcare disciplines that interact with nursing. As healthcare continues to change, new roles are cropping up, and historical roles are being redefined. And all of these changes come with students. The staff educator must understand these roles in order to educate the nurse learner. For example, as healthcare continues to move to more and more care being provided outside acute care hospitals, the role of the medical assistant continues to expand. Can the RN delegate to the medical assistant in your state and within your facility?

Other expanding roles with which the educator must be familiar in order to provide the nurse learner with the knowledge required to work with them in the clinical settings include behavioral or mental health specialists, care navigators, and care or case managers.

Communication and Nursing Professional Development

Communication is an important aspect to ensuring the nurse learner understands the rationale for change and can subsequently implement the change. In addition, communication is a critical piece to promoting a healthy environment, which is why it is listed here in the overview of the nursing professional development specialist's role. The staff educator needs to consider communication, essentially marketing, by being knowledgeable about which of the following to use (as well as when and why to use them):

- Informatics
- Technology
- Social or collaborative learning, including gamification and mobile learning
- Social media
- Current awareness specific to the educator

Subsequent chapters include additional information about these communication topics.

Conclusion

With the broad education goals of transferring learning to behavior and demonstrating the value of education, the nursing professional development specialist must use influence, resources, and networking to ensure the goals are met. In many ways, by maintaining competence in the field of nursing professional development, staff educators provide the nursing profession with nurse learners who are striving to lead change by advancing the health of the people.

Florence Nightingale once said,

Nursing is an art: and if it is to be made an art, it requires an exclusive devotion as hard a preparation, as any painter's or sculptor's work; for what is the having to do with dead canvas or dead marble, compared with having to do with the living body, the temple of God's spirit? It is one of the Fine Arts: I had almost said, the finest of Fine Arts.

Although the professional development specialist's role continues to focus on its roots of orientation, inservicing, CE, and student services, it has expanded to include education being an integral part of:

- Quality improvement, EBP, and research to generate new knowledge for the practice of education

- Certification of RNs

- Magnet and shared governance for those who are on that journey

And who knows what continued changes the role might begin to see in the future.

Questions for Reflection/Discussion

1. Could you teach nursing practice differently depending upon the content? Assess differently? Evaluate differently?

2. Where are your "think spots"—your learning spaces? For example, do you want to promote collaboration? How do you (or could you) provide venues for asynchronous and synchronous discussions?

3. Do you use the Socratic method to reinforce learning? For example, do you develop questions such as "Can you explain what is happening..." or "What other way would you plan to...?"

4. Have you worked with leadership to develop a standard method of providing feedback to colleagues?

KEY TAKEAWAYS

- *Know that as a nursing professional development specialist you are responsible for a variety of tasks.*
- *Recognize that you are responsible for your own growth and development in many areas.*

Resources

American Nurses Association. (2014). Professional role competence. Retrieved from http://www.nursingworld.org/MainMenuCategories/ThePracticeofProfessionalNursing/NursingStandards/Professional-Role-Competence.html

The Joint Commission. (2004). Preventing infant death and injury during delivery. *Sentinel Event Alert*, (30). Retrieved from http://www.jointcommission.org/sentinel_event_alert_issue_30_preventing_infant_death_and_injury_during_delivery/

The Joint Commission. (2008). Preventing pediatric medication errors. *Sentinel Event Alert*, (39). Retrieved from http://www.jointcommission.org/sentinel_event_alert_issue_39_preventing_pediatric_medication_errors/

References

American Nurses Association & National Nursing Staff Development Organization. (2010). *Nursing professional development: Scope and standards of practice.* Silver Spring, MD: American Nurses Association.

Benner, P. (1984). *From novice to expert: Excellence and power in clinical nursing practice.* Menlo Park, CA: Addison-Wesley.

Institute for Healthcare Improvement. (2015). IHI Triple Aim initiative. Retrieved from http://www.ihi.org/engage/initiatives/TripleAim/Pages/default.aspx

Institute of Medicine. (2003). *Health profession education: A bridge to quality* (pp. 45–74). Washington, DC: National Academies Press.

Institute of Medicine. (2010). *The future of nursing: Leading change, advancing health.* Washington, DC: National Academies Press. Retrieved from http://www.iom.edu/Reports/2010/The-Future-of-Nursing-Leading-Change-Advancing-Health.aspx

Interprofessional Education Collaborative Expert Panel. (2011). *Core competencies for interprofessional collaborative practice: Report of an expert panel.* Washington, DC: Interprofessional Education Collaborative.

Kirkpatrick, D. L., & Kirkpatrick, J. D. (2005). *Transferring learning to behavior: Using the four levels to improve performance.* San Francisco, CA: Berrett-Koehler.

McCrindle, M. (2015). Generation Z characteristics. (Blog). Retrieved from http://generationz.com.au/characteristics/

Mueller, J. (2015). Generation Z characteristics. Retrieved from http://www.ehow.com/info_8056211_generation-characteristics.html

National League for Nursing. (2012). *Outcomes and competencies for graduates of practical/vocational, diploma, baccalaureate, master's practice doctorate, and research doctorate programs in nursing.* Washington, DC: Author.

Patterson, K., Grenny, J., Maxfield, D., McMillan, R., & Switzler, A. (2008). *Influencer: The power to change anything.* New York, NY: McGraw-Hill.

QSEN Institute. (2014). *Competencies.* Retrieved from http://qsen.org/competencies/

Shah, R. (2011). Working with five generations in the workplace. *Forbes.* Retrieved from http://www.forbes.com/sites/rawnshah/2011/04/20/working-with-five-generations-in-the-workplace/

Tauber, T., & Johnson, D. (2014). Meet the modern learner. (Infographic). Bersin by Deloitte. Retrieved from http://www.bersin.com/Practice/Detail.aspx?id=18071

CHAPTER 2

Analyzing the Need for Professional Development Activities

Introduction

Chapter 1 briefly introduced the ADDIE model; this chapter focuses on the model's first step: Analysis. Analyzing (or assessing) a problem, issue, situation, need, or gap is always the first component of working toward a solution. The analysis phase could occur when a regulatory body communicates a new practice requirement (for example, The Joint Commission annually releases the updated National Patient Safety Goals). Why? Because there may be a gap that education can fulfill between the current practice and the new required practice. Or this phase could require a month (or more) of work with focus groups and individual interviews—the actual length depends on how long it takes to understand the root of your problem. Although you might not always have the time and resources to do an ideal analysis of the situation (also known as a *needs assessment*), the more fully you understand the problem, the better equipped you will be to work toward a solution. Anybody could begin the process of problem identification, but it is the staff educator who is responsible for performing a complete analysis that initiates the formal ADDIE sequence.

We have organized the needs assessment into six major components, which follow the order of the discussion in this chapter. In practice, however, you're likely to move back and forth between these steps:

1. Begin a formal analysis process.

2. Identify key stakeholders.

3. Foster stakeholder ownership.

4. Perform the needs assessment.

5. Present the results of the needs assessment.

6. Determine the plan of action for the proposed education (see Chapter 3, "Designing and Developing Professional Development Activities").

> **NOTE**
>
> *A professional development activity is the response to a problem, issue, situation, need, or gap. Anecdotally, different parts of the country use different terms. In this chapter, we refer to all of these events that result in a professional development activity simply as a "need."*

Beginning the Analysis Process

Within the context of nursing professional development activities, a *needs assessment* is a process of identifying the gap between an existing condition and a desired condition. We have to work hard to get at the root cause(s) of the problem. When someone states the problem, ask, "If we fix that, would we still have the problem?" This question helps to eliminate the symptoms as well as determine if the problem is one of learner accountability. If the problem involves knowledge, behavior, or skill, education is likely to help. If the problem involves the supporting environment—data, resources, systems—then there is a management component that must be addressed.

Educational Needs Versus System Problems

An *educational need* represents a gap or deficiency between the learners' present level of competency and a higher level required for effective performance. What is the existing condition/competency and the desired condition/level of competency? For example, The Joint Commission publishes the National Patient Safety Goals (TJC, 2015) related to various areas of healthcare safety. One goal is to prevent infection, and the TJC recommendation is to follow hand-cleaning guidelines from the Centers for Disease Control and Prevention. Facilities are asked to set goals to improve compliance rates. Here, the needs assessment focuses on a gap analysis of an existing condition (80% compliance rate; recent increase in nosocomial infections) versus the desired condition (100% compliance rate for following hand-washing guidelines; decrease in nosocomial infections).

There can be four levels of need: professional, individual, community, and organizational/departmental. Let's say the organization needs to move from Point A (current condition) to Point B (desired condition), as in the example where an organization is not Magnet certified (Point A, current condition) but desires to become Magnet certified (Point B, desired condition). Taking this example further, at the professional level, as more organizations become Magnet certified, the desired condition of more satisfied nurses and better patient care is reached. At the community level, more patients are cared for in Magnet certified facilities. At the individual level, more learners are certified in their specialty (desired condition) as part of the organization's journey to become Magnet certified.

When the focus of the gap is the individual, the resulting educational need can be one of knowledge and/or interest to the individual learner, can be related to a new required skill, or can be a desired behavior change. It is often difficult to get at the root causes of the problem, and investigating which domain of learning (that is, cognitive, psychomotor, or affective) is predominantly the reason for the gap helps the staff educator and manager discover whether education might be the answer. Sometimes, the problem can be fixed through review of the expectations of accountability, or it can be a combination of both education delivery and accountability assurance. It is why the gap must be analyzed through a needs assessment because not infrequently, when stakeholders state there is a problem, they are likely stating a symptom of an underlying problem.

For the purposes of professional development, a stakeholder is anyone who delivers, facilitates, or receives professional nursing care. Stakeholders include but are not limited to direct care providing nurses, nurse managers, staff educators, executive leadership, patients, and families.

One key question to keep handy during a needs assessment is, "If we fix [fill in the blank], would we still have the problem?" This question can help staff educators and managers differentiate between *symptoms* and *system problems*. In addition, the answer helps educators and managers know whether to define the issue as either of the following:

- A *system problem* (involving the supporting facts, including data, resources, or incentives), which management needs to address prior to investing the resources to educate or re-educate staff

- An *educational need* (involving the learner's knowledge, skill, or behavior), where management and the educator work together to educate or re-educate staff as the first course of action to solve the problem

DISCRIMINATING BETWEEN SYSTEM PROBLEMS AND EDUCATIONAL NEEDS

Take a moment to read through the following scenarios, which illustrate the difference between a system problem and an educational need.

Scenario 1: *Nurse manager Mike comes to your office stating that many staff members are not documenting that patient baths were provided during a shift. He requests that you put together a learning activity to cover appropriate documentation standards. You ask, "If we educate staff, would we still have the problem?" In this case, you know that the electronic health record had recently undergone major revisions, and the location for documenting patient baths is no longer in the nurses' most commonly used flow sheets. Instead of re-educating staff members, you suggest to Mike that he ask the informatics team to reconsider placement of this documentation piece because this gap sounds more like a system problem rather than an educational need.*

Scenario 2: *Clinical director Dinah comes to your office stating that there have been several patient care errors surrounding use of a new patient lift device. As Dinah explains more about the errors to you, you begin to realize that no training has been provided to the nurses or* *physical therapists on how to use this new equipment. In asking, "If we educate staff, would we still have the problem?" you answer, "Hopefully not." This gap sounds more like an educational need than a system problem (well, except for the system problem concerning how new equipment was introduced without someone notifying the educator!).*

In identifying the difference between an educational need and a system problem, the staff educator may work alone or in conjunction with a manager.

Education Problems Versus Management Problems

After determining that the problem is not (completely) a management issue, the staff educator is responsible for working with the manager to determine the framework for when the answer lies partly in the education or re-education of staff. This task is the second step of the needs assessment.

> **NOTE**
>
> *If the manager fulfills the role of the educator, then the responsibility for both education and learner accountability lies within the educator's purview.*

The following example illustrates the educator's responsibility for determining the education versus management issue:

The nurse learners have been educated on a new policy stating the need for patient reassessment post intervention (medication, repositioning, and so on) along with appropriate documentation of these actions. The educator has ensured all staff are aware of the policy and the date for implementation. Essentially, the educator thinks the distribution of this new policy statement is merely a for-your-information (FYI) notice— there shouldn't be a need for specific education. Yet when the educator reviews the data 2 months after the policy change, the unit has only a 70% implementation rate.

NOTE

In the preceding example, the organization should determine what the percentage completion rate is for learner education, expected date for implementation, and consequences for not implementing. You can work with the safety and compliance staff to be sure you are aware of the expected rates of completion and compliance. Although the Centers for Medicare and Medicaid Services' implementation requirements are fondly known as the "all or none club"—where compliance is defined as 100% of all patients, all the time—the organization demonstrates to The Joint Commission how the organization is meeting/working toward the required standards. For example, the organization implemented a specific educational program that decreased the amount of surgical site infections by 10%.

To determine the next steps, the educator needs to ask the following:

1. Was the required percentage of staff educated on the policy expectations by the implementation date? If yes, proceed to Question 2. If no, determine who fell off the bus (for example, learners on a specific shift).

2. Were there specific points of the policy that were not implemented? If yes, then the educator knows where to focus the re-education. In our example, perhaps documentation is lacking. If so, then documentation examples can be provided.

3. Why are the nurses not documenting? The educator should make a point to ask nurse learners this question in person. If the educator is unable to do so, the educator can place a large piece of paper in the break room and ask nurses to note their reasons for not documenting. In doing so, the educator will find out if the managers need to address other issues, such as whether specific learners struggle with all documentation or all forms of change.

The key is to teach the learners how to integrate the expectation of any policy into their daily practice. Quite simply, it is through practice and reinforcement daily. (For more information, you might consider reading *The Power of Habit* [Duhigg, 2014].) For the nurse learner in this situation, the documentation examples could be part of a huddle (during a brief group meeting at shift change) for a week. Then during the next week's huddle, the educator or charge nurse asks those in attendance for specific examples related to the policy. Something as simple as this huddle also provides learners with the understanding that they own their practice, as the educator appeals to their caring nature and adult learning principles.

"WHEN EVERYONE IS RESPONSIBLE"

Let's consider an example where patients have a problem with skin redness and irritation. Because the Centers for Medicare and Medicaid Services classify pressure ulcers as a "never event" (AHRQ, 2014), does this mean only the RN staff have the responsibility for identifying and documenting the potential for the development of a pressure ulcer? No.

Patients, regardless of the setting in which they are cared for, are the responsibility of whichever discipline happens to be providing care at any given time. The occupational and physical therapy staff who are working with a patient and see an area of redness under a compression boot are responsible for documenting and notifying the RN. As the coordinator of care, it is the RN's responsibility to follow up and develop a plan of care. Teamwork is one of the Institute of Medicine's interprofessional care competencies, and the example is teamwork in action (IOM, 2003).

A Framework for Education

The staff educator and manager are responsible for developing the framework for education and conveying its importance of fostering professional development within the context of the framework. The manager acts to demonstrate the alignment of:

- The organization's strategic plan
- Goals of the discipline of nursing, such as elevation of nursing practice through shared governance or the Magnet journey
- Nursing philosophy of the unit/area/organization
- Outside forces, such as regulatory agency requirements or IOM reports
- Quality, safety, and performance improvement work
- A focus on the manager's area of responsibility along the continuum of a specific patient population

Creating a visual of all the components and posting them in an area visible to all staff assists individual nurse learners in valuing and applying to their own practice the learnings from each professional development activity in which they participate.

Use of a visual allows the staff educator to draw the link for staff between the nursing professional development activities within the context of the strategic goals of the organization, unit or area, and even specific patient population. The educator's goal is to tie learning to strategy, leadership message, accountability, and measurement. To achieve this goal, the educators actually have their own product line, and the learning activities tie the line together. By *product line* we mean learning activities that are part of a professional development program for educators themselves. For example, the educator who works for an organization that has several educators may have developed a standardized means of how to communicate policy and procedure changes. Thus, regardless of where educators work, the standardized communication plan can be used and is seen as a component of an educator's product line. The components include the following:

- Patient (individual) and/or patient population
- Area of practice or specific overall product line (GI, surgery, cardiology, and so on)
- Staff (nurse/all disciplines)
- Manager expectations
- Department or business unit (such as Nursing or Patient Services)
- Facility's strategic plan

For example, imagine that upon completion of the analysis phase of the need, it has been determined that education will assist in solving the problem identified as "increase in readmissions of femur fracture patients due to infection." Here is a simple way for the staff educator to frame the learning activity that needs to be designed:

- Patient = Femur fracture
- Area of practice = Ambulatory clinic
- Staff = Medical assistant and/or RN

- Manager expectations = Decrease the number of admissions by $x\%$, resulting in cost savings and improved *National Database of Nursing Quality Indicators* (NDNQI) scores

- Department/business unit = Orthopedics

- Facility's strategic plan = Meet the Institute for Healthcare Improvement Triple Aim of decreased cost, increased quality, and patient engagement (IHI, 2015)

Identifying Stakeholders

After determining that education is necessary to fulfill the need, the staff educator and manager must work together to define which staff members to educate. Often, all members of the healthcare team must be educated on a particular subject, whether it's simply at the level of awareness or at the level of responsibility for implementation and evaluation.

To begin this process, the staff educator needs to identify which staff roles are involved in all aspects of the need. (The people who fill these roles are known as *stakeholders*.) In other words, who is affected both upstream and downstream by the situation? By identifying all the stakeholders, the staff educator ensures every perspective is taken into account. Including all perspectives leads to a determination of where the scope of accountability lies—either with the management structure or the education of the staff, and, more often than not, both the educator and manager own at least a portion of the responsibility. The responsibility for participating in the nursing professional development activities and subsequent application of the learning is that of the individual learner.

Fostering Stakeholder Ownership

Now we know this *never* happens, but on the off chance you have any learners who are less than pleased with an upcoming continuing education (CE) activity, consider the following:

- Educators are really in sales, using the art of persuasion and, in essence, being the consummate influencer. The role is all about appealing to the educator's lifelong learner colleagues. (Although a gentle reminder to colleagues that being a professional healthcare provider comes with lifelong learning is sometimes helpful, make sure that the message doesn't come across with a demeaning tone.)

- Selling is the art of reading and persuading people: Know your learning activity or educational program thoroughly, be confident in why and how the learning will help the learner and the patient, and, above all, think like the learner. Selling is not about logic, but emotions. Selling the activity transfers ownership of the content that is then applied at the bedside.

Consider the following when "selling" CE activities:

- **Adult learning principles.** What does the learner already know about the content of the planned continuing education activity? Can you share with the learner the rationale for the requirement? How can you incorporate the preferred learning methods of the learners?

- **Influencer model components.** As outlined in the book *Influencer* (Patterson, Grenny, Maxfield, McMillan, & Switzler, 2008), consider all components in terms of how the staff educator "sells" the implementation phase of the activity. If the activity focuses on updating a skill, based on the model, the educator will want to understand the learners (personal motivation/ability), the unit/area of practice (social motivation/ability), and the facility (structural motivation/ability). See Table 2.1.

  For example, if there are new regulations regarding how blood is to be administered, the educator needs to know how much the learner knows about blood administration, and whether the learners have experience administering blood (personal). The educator uses the more experienced learner RNs to educate or role model the updated procedure (social). The educator has evaluation requirements such as tracking education/follow-up data to ensure the learner is successful and the procedure is a success (structural).

TABLE 2.1   *PERSONAL, SOCIAL, AND STRUCTURAL APPLICATIONS FOR ENSURING STAKEHOLDER OWNERSHIP*

APPLICATION	MOTIVATION	ABILITY
Personal What is the experience of the nurse with administering blood?	Make the undesirable desirable.	Surpass your limits.
Social Has the preceptor reviewed the current policy/procedure?	Harness peer pressure.	Find strength in numbers.
Structural What process does the educator have in place for how frequently the competency is reviewed and how the competency is tracked?	Design rewards and demand accountability.	Change the environment.

After you have identified and engaged your stakeholders, you can start collecting data from them. There are actually two types of data you can collect with a needs assessment: qualitative (subjective) and quantitative (objective). In the world of needs assessments, the *qualitative data* is gathered from the questions you ask of people, whereas the *quantitative data* is gathered from the questions you ask while observing and/or measuring processes and outcomes.

Gathering Qualitative Data

Following are some examples of common questions to ask of the various stakeholders for a subjective needs assessment:

- What new or continuous problems do you face?
- What new procedures, equipment or initiatives affect your area?
- Do you have data from incident reports, patient or staff surveys, or performance improvement reports that indicate that a problem exists?

In asking these questions of stakeholders, the professional development specialist receives qualitative data that can be reviewed for themes. Themes that are common among the various stakeholders can be validated in the available quantitative data. Consider developing a set of critical thinking questions that are specific to the work setting. By using any of the six levels of Bloom's taxonomy (knowledge, comprehension, application, analysis, synthesis, or evaluation) and the three domains of learning (cognitive, psychomotor, and affective), the staff educator can build a simple and effective needs assessment to get a qualitative baseline of any intended professional development activity (McDonald, 2013).

> **NOTE**
>
> One current theme that is being discussed at all levels of healthcare organizations is patient experience (satisfaction). On the one hand, the patient experience is a goal of the IHI Triple Aim. On the other hand, data noting the patient experience theme can be found in patient satisfaction survey results, discussion with staff on the most common issues and requests from patients and their families, and even the number of referrals to the organization regarding specific surgeries.

If there is an issue with a change in practice, such as the implementation of a new infusion pump, the educator can follow up with additional, positive questions that address the practice change, such as those from the following list. In the case of the first two questions, the educator would include words, such as "infusion pumps," that more specifically describe the issue:

- What is the biggest problem you… (are having with the infusion pumps)?
- What is preventing you from… (using the infusion pumps)?
- What type of help do you need?
- How are you impacted by this problem?
- Who else do you see impacted by this problem (for example, other staff, patients, or families)?
- Do you believe education can solve this problem? (If not, what do you see as potential solutions?)

Gathering Quantitative Data

The staff educator then validates the information gleaned from the stakeholders through a review of the available hard or quantitative data. Such actual evidence does exist and is used as the objective portion of the needs assessment. Many times, however, the staff educator is unaware of the location of the data or exactly what comprises the data. In these situations, the manager (line leader) and educator (informal leader) must *share* knowledge for the greater good of both staff and patients. You can find quantitative evidence internally, and it is often benchmarked externally through such groups as NDNQI (http://nursingworld.org/Research-Toolkit/NDNQI), Leapfrog (www.leapfroggroup.org), Agency for Healthcare Research and Quality (AHRQ; www.ahrq.gov), The Joint Commission (www.jointcommission.org), and the Centers for Medicare and Medicaid Services (www.cms.gov).

FOR THOSE NEW TO THE STAFF EDUCATOR ROLE

If the preceding abbreviations and sources of quantitative/objective data seem a little foreign to you, it will be well worth your time to gain a working familiarity with them. You want to explore both the publically available websites as well as your organization's internal data. The websites include information such as aggregate benchmarks of multiple organizations, the purpose behind measuring certain indicators, definitions of each measure, and even toolkits for making improvement.

In contrast, the people and data sources affiliated with these reports inside your organization give you an idea of your specific organization's performance. Building relationships with the people in this department helps you get access to the data when you need it, be familiar with organizational priorities (especially if you're in a larger organization), and gain access to experts who understand this data quite well.

Sharing the Value of the Education With Learners

It is important for the educator to post a visual noting how the professional development activity that results from a needs assessment actually affects the care provided. If the learner does not understand the value of the education, the learner will not apply the knowledge, skill, or desired behavior.

How does the staff educator help the learner value the education as well as his or her role? Sometimes it's as simple as the staff educator providing the rationale for the change (that is, explaining how the change affects patient care, such as outcomes, experience, or decreased cost). Those in the nursing profession must understand they "own" care. How the nurse learner practices is what predominantly affects the success of accountable care, the Triple Aim, whether the facility meets targets (such as decreases in readmission rates), whether the facility goals are met, and whether both the nurse and patient are satisfied.

The value to the nurse learner lies in his or her ability to understand that the role as a patient advocate begins with how the nurse practices on a daily basis.

Performing a Needs Assessment

After the stakeholders have been identified, and the staff educator develops a subjective needs assessment and gathers the corresponding objective evidence, the next step is to choose one or more methods to assess the problem. Recall that a needs assessment or gap analysis can focus on several of the four levels at one time: professional, community, individual, or organization.

What's the goal for the needs assessment? Is it all-encompassing, such as "competent, confident caregivers?" If so, how will the needs assessment be measured? As Stephen Covey (1989) states, "Begin with the end in mind."

A needs assessment typically produces two lists: a list of problems education will fix and a list of problems managers can fix. Ultimately, these lists provide the rationale for why managers and educators must be on the same page. In all actuality, depending upon how long the issue has existed, the solution will contain both elements of education and accountability for practice.

Needs may be identified within a variety of concerns related to your unit, department, or workplace, such as the following:

- Current problems and issues

- Future problems and issues

- General industry needs

- Needs in specialized areas

- Needs arising from change

- Social, economic, political concerns

- Job performance

- Thematic or programmatic areas

The following are some reasons for conducting a needs assessment:

- Identifying the present situation (never taking it at face value, ask the questions).

- Determining how the current situation differs from the desired situation. What are the parameters?

- Finding out who is affected. Take a vertical slice of the organization when doing a needs assessment; don't necessarily work from the top down.

- Assessing the organizational climate.

Now that we've covered some of the overarching principles and the who and what of a needs assessment, let's start talking about *how* you actually go about completing a needs assessment. Tools of a needs assessment include:

- Observations

- Questionnaires

- Consultations

- Work samples/task analysis

- Focus groups/appreciative inquiry

- Self-assessments/tests

- Data

- Strengths, weakness, opportunities, threats (SWOT)

- Failure modes and effects analysis (FMEA)

Observations

The nurse educator who is focused on teaching either a new procedure skill or a revision to an existing procedure skill uses observations as the gold standard. In the case of teaching a new procedure skill, the educator observes the skill as currently being performed and compares it with the updated version. Consider observations on off-shift as well as weekends. For example, what if your rate of urinary tract infections has increased? Use the procedure checklist and observe a few learners, and note any trends or procedure steps not being followed.

Questionnaires

Questionnaires are used when the focus is on disseminating new knowledge to the learner; they should also be used as part of assessing a skill because the nurse learner needs to understand the rationale for the change. Use open-ended questions designed to elicit information that will assist the educator to develop and design the education that meets the intended outcomes. For example, if there is an issue with "patient falls," begin with knowledge questions related to the learner's knowledge of what is required to implement the facility's policy with regard to this problem. Many times, learners aren't aware of the expectations because communication regarding policy changes may be lacking. (It's sad to say, but sometimes your practice is only as good as the day you began due to the human condition of fear of change!)

Consultations

The educator might often feel like he or she is the last to know about an upcoming change that affects the specific work area or patient population. If so, the educator can take a more proactive stance and meet on a regular basis with the manager to discuss upcoming initiatives. Create a standardized form in order to be able to note your progress, the progress of education, and upcoming work. You could even develop and use a scorecard for these meetings.

Work Samples/Task Analysis

Similar to observation, work samples/task analysis are taken a step further and used when revising and validating the role of learners and follow-up education for the role. An old, well-known method is Developing a Curriculum (DACUM). The educator works with a group of 10 to 12 experts to create the task analysis by:

1. Using a written description of the role (RN, LPN, MA)

2. Identifying general areas of competence

3. Identifying specific skills and structuring skills into learning

4. Establishing competence for each skill

In using the DACUM method for job analysis, educators and managers need to work together to ensure specifics for all roles that can be seen as infringing upon the practice of nursing (and there are many).

Focus Groups/Appreciative Inquiry

Staff educators may choose to use focus groups as a means of assessing what various stakeholders find to be issues. Develop five or six questions related to the issue, use and follow the agenda, stick to the time on the agenda, and either have someone take notes or record the session. In many ways, depending upon how the educator uses focus groups, it is a form of action research known as *appreciative inquiry*. It is one way to engage the learner in the ADDIE process itself and results in ownership of the desired change.

Self-Assessment or Tests

Self-assessment or tests are important to needs assessment, but they are not normally performed due to the lack of a standardized self-assessment pertinent to the topic or the educator's lack of time to generate one. That said, the staff educator should consider having all staff members complete the online VARK (visual, aural, read/write, kinesthetic) assessment so the educator knows the predominant learning preferences of staff members. Knowing learning preferences of staff members assists the educator in the development and design phases.

It might also assist the staff educator in matching newly hired staff members with preceptors. You can use the free tool at http://vark-learn. com/the-vark-questionnaire.

Data

Data is comparing internal data specific to the educator's area with external benchmarked data across a patient population or a specific type of healthcare environment, such as the ambulatory setting. (Check out the "For Those New to the Staff Educator Role" feature earlier in this chapter for more information.)

INSERVICE EXAMPLE

The staff educator learned of the following information from the ECRI Institute (Emergency Care Research Institute) patient safety organization website (www.ecri.org): "For the fourth year in a row, clinical alarm hazards, a Joint Commission National Patient Safety Goal, remains number one on ECRI's list. Alarm hazards, electronic health record data integrity issues, and infusion line mix-ups top the list." There is also information from The Joint Commission noting how to manage the risk of tubing misconnections while manufacturers work toward standardizing all tubing connectors:

- *What is the responsibility of the educator now knowledgeable of these topics?*
- *Has there been an issue in the past at the educator's facility?*
- *Has the facility made the necessary changes to standard tubing?*
- *Does the facility have standards for alarm settings? Integration with the electronic medical record (EMR)?*

Going through these types of Analysis questions allows the educator to determine whether a simple communication is warranted, or, in the event the facility hasn't standardized tubing, whether the simple communication should include visuals of what connector goes with what tubing or where the learner can find the information (or both).

SWOT

Strengths, weaknesses, opportunities, and threats (SWOT) of the potential issue/problem are generated/reviewed. SWOT is an assessment often used in conjunction with committees or focus groups. The educator uses a large sheet of paper (or similar medium) with space for each of the four components. The educator can act as a facilitator who works through SWOT. Alternatively, you may choose to split the group into sections who participate in a round-robin discussion and then get back together as one group to review.

FMEA

Failure modes and effects analysis (FMEA) is often used to determine what has happened when there has been an error or to think proactively through how an error might occur. It is an objective way of determining what occurred and what steps to take to prevent an error from happening in the future. If you're new to FMEA, an online search of "FMEA templates" should help you find one that works for you.

Presenting the Results of the Needs Assessment

When the professional development specialist has collected the needs assessment data, it's time to circle back and present the findings to the stakeholders. Hopefully, the staff educator has determined upfront whether only the findings are being presented or the findings *and* potential education plan are being presented concurrently. For example, if the facility has shared governance committees representing the staff (learner) aspect of practice (education, care, research, and evidence), the educator would certainly include these stakeholders in viewing the findings of the analysis. Similarly, the educator would include managers and all other groups of stakeholders.

The focus of the presentation becomes the *what* and *how* by which the findings are to be presented. You'll also want to consider what to do if there is push back to the findings or to the plan. Because the evidence shows there is too much information for people to process at any given time (*The Economist*, 2011), simply going to a meeting and giving a slide presentation is not sufficient to deliver the most effective message. Always include a one-page document of the essence of the findings, potential education plan, and how the education will be implemented and evaluated. In fact, going to a meeting might not be in the best interest of stakeholders if the impending education is not up for discussion. It is the staff educator who knows the learners and facility best and should work toward developing a *standardized* plan for how to present the findings of the needs assessment (gap analysis) to the various groups of stakeholders.

Conclusion

The importance of conducting a formal needs assessment to begin the ADDIE sequence cannot be understated. Not only will rigorously exploring the need ensure you can resolve the need with a learning activity, but it also provides you with baseline data you will need when performing the evaluation step following the learning activity. We hope the variety of techniques for performing a needs assessment have added to your educator toolkit and that you get comfortable with several, but don't forget to branch out from time to time (there is no one-size-fits-all approach to performing the Analysis phase of the ADDIE model, so feel free to get creative!). Whichever tool you choose, we guarantee you that taking the time to complete this first step will save you much time in the long run.

Questions for Reflection/Discussion

1. Who are the key stakeholders in your organization, and how can they contribute to a needs assessment?

2. What are the primary sources of quantitative/objective data available to you, and how might you get access to more of these sources?

3. What needs assessment techniques seem most easy (and most challenging) to you?

4. What are some strategies you could employ to help learners find greater value in education?

KEY TAKEAWAYS

- *Performing a needs assessment is absolutely necessary for successful professional development activities.*
- *Identifying and engaging the key stakeholders at the beginning of the Analysis phase helps to facilitate adequate data collection.*
- *Both qualitative and quantitative data are beneficial for a complete needs assessment.*

> • *A variety of needs assessment tools are available, and selection can depend on tool familiarity, context of the need/organization, and resource availability.*

Resources

Duhigg, C. (2014). *The power of habit: Why we do what we do in life and business*. New York, NY: Random House.

References

Agency for Healthcare Research and Quality. (2014). Never events. Retrieved from https://www.cms.gov/Newsroom/MediaReleaseDatabase/Press-releases/2009-Press-releases-items/2009-01-153.html

Covey, S. R. (1989). *Seven habits of highly effective people.* New York, NY: Simon & Schuster.

The Economist. (2011, June 30). Too much information [Web log post]. Retrieved from http://www.economist.com/node/18895468

Institute for Healthcare Improvement. (2015). The IHI triple aim. Retrieved from http://www.ihi.org/engage/initiatives/TripleAim/Pages/default.aspx

Institute of Medicine. (2003). *Health profession education: A bridge to quality*. Washington, DC: National Academies Press.

The Joint Commission. (2015). National patient safety goals. Retrieved from www.jointcommission.org/assets/1/6/2015_HAP_NPSG_ER.pdf

McDonald, M. (2013). *The nurse educator's guide to assessing learning outcomes.* Burlington, MA: Jones & Bartlett.

Patterson, K., Grenny, J., Maxfield, D., McMillan, R., & Switzler, A. (2008). *Influencer: The power to change anything.* New York, NY: McGraw-Hill.

CHAPTER 3

Designing and Developing Professional Development Activities

Introduction

At this point, you have established the need for one or more professional development activities, and you have stakeholders on board who confirm the need really is a need that could be addressed with education. It's now time for step 2 of the ADDIE model: designing and developing your learning activity so that it addresses those needs identified in the analysis phase. To do this, we encourage you to leverage beneficial learning theories and models, recognize your organization's resources and limitations, and continue to engage key stakeholders. We begin this chapter by walking you through these components, and conclude with useful strategies for the educator to use that will assist the learners in integrating the new knowledge/skill/ behavior from these educational activities into their daily practice.

Learning Theories and Models

Although you might be thinking that the consideration of learning theories and models is a waste of time, we have yet to meet a professional development specialist who doesn't quickly see value in using some of these theories or models to guide their practice in the professional development role. The practice of education is a bit different from the practice of clinical nursing, making some additional guidance quite beneficial. And that's our perspective on learning theories and models: They serve as a beneficial guide. They're not something you have to commit to memory; rather, they're something that you learn to use and apply almost naturally.

Staff educators who have an awareness of the current learning theories and models can choose to commit to using one when designing educational programs, or they can review the options and choose a theory or model based upon the desired outcome of the learning activity or education program. (That is, in theory!) What often happens, however, is educators may not have any academic preparation in learning theories and models, or they might not think to search and use the evidence on what theories and models are being used in nursing practice as they design educational programs.

To address those issues, we start this section by demonstrating how learning theories and models are categorized, beginning with paradigms. A *paradigm* is a distinct concept or thought pattern, and notes specific theories and models an author uses. Then we provide you with an inclusive list of these learning theories and models, as well as additional information such as applications, principles, and examples for each.

> **NOTE**
>
> *The Learning Theories website (http://www.learning-theories.com) contains details of several learning theories and models about how people learn.*

Nursing's Metaparadigm

The metaparadigm (*meta* being Greek for "that which is behind") for the nursing profession consists of person, health, environment, and nursing. It is the role of the staff educator to frame all content of the educational component being designed within the context of nursing's metaparadigm. Why? The four components of nursing's metaparadigm can assist the educator with ensuring the content is incorporated into the learner's practice of nursing.

> **NOTE**
>
> Per Oxford Dictionaries ("paradigm," 2015), the technical definition of *paradigm* is "a typical example or pattern of something." Synonyms of paradigm include *model, pattern, example, exemplar, template,* and *standard.* Look at the synonyms and consider how, as educators design and develop the education, the educators are responsible for seeing the big picture for the nurse learner by being aware of the paradigms and knowledgeable about the learning theories.

One way to ensure that you always include the nursing metaparadigm in the creation of continuing education (CE) activities is to ask additional Analysis questions (see Table 3.1); the answers will inform the Design phase of meeting a learning need. Why do this? Because you (as well as the manager) should have the most clear-cut picture of the overall nursing practice expected in your area.

Asking questions like those shown in Table 3.1 is like being situationally aware and mindful of what is taking place with your patient. This situational awareness is a key component of keeping patients safe. And it is the nurse as a lifelong learner who is the patient's first and last line of defense.

> **NOTE**
>
> Although this chapter focuses on learning theories used in developing/designing nursing education for the nurse learner, two books the educator should read to inform implementation of education are Clinical Wisdom and Interventions in Acute and Critical Care (Benner, Hooper Kyriakidis, & Stannard, 2011) and The Power of Habit (Duhigg, 2014).

TABLE 3.1   *NURSING METAPARADIGM AND IMPLICATIONS*

METAPARADIGM COMPONENT	QUESTIONS TO ASK	IMPLICATIONS
Person	What are the expectations of the nurse for educating the patient and family as a result of the learning activity?	There is *always* education the nurse should include, whether he or she is learning new information, taking on a new task, or addressing a change in behavior. How else will the nursing profession meet the recommendations of the Institute for Healthcare Improvement (IHI, 2015) Triple Aim (patient engagement) and the 2010 Institute of Medicine (IOM) report "The Future of Nursing: Leading Change, Advancing Health" that "Nurses should be full partners, with physicians and other health professionals, in redesigning health care in the United States" (p. 1)?
Health	What other healthcare professionals need to be aware of the proposed changes that are to result from the learning activity?	If other healthcare professionals, such as Respiratory Therapists, are to reinforce the change, shouldn't they be included in the education, or at least be given a "cheat sheet" of the change and consequent expectations? This is where having knowledge of learning theories and models comes into play. If the academicians are teaching "interprofessionally," shouldn't those educators in practice settings continue the path? How else will you change healthcare? (Yet, please remember it is the *nurse* who is the *coordinator* of care. As other professional roles are expanding and changing and often do not include nursing, the area of *care coordination* cannot be given up!)

Environment	What physical concepts need a reminder (for example, infection control principles such as hand washing)? What are the cultural/diversity aspects that need to be taken into account?	Has your facility adopted a cultural/diversity model such as the one published in the article "The Process of Cultural Competence in the Delivery of Healthcare Services: A Model of Care" (Campinha-Bacote, 2002)? Or does your facility use the National Standards for Culturally and Linguistically Appropriate Services in Health and Health Care (National CLAS Standards), which can be found at https://www.thinkculturalhealth.hhs. gov/content/clas.asp? The National Association of School Nurses Cultural Competency Assessment Checklist (http:// www.nasn.org/ToolsResources/CulturalCompetency/ CulturalCompetencyAssessmentChecklist) incorporates the principles of cultural competence by asking, "Tell me about your...." Such a question helps the learners understand how to incorporate the content they have learned and apply it to the individual patient.
Nursing	What "caring" aspects of nursing can be added to the continuing education (CE) activity? What behaviors separate nursing care from other professions?	It's easy to forget the reasons for practicing nursing; behaviors specific to nursing are to be reiterated in all programs. It could be as simple as reminding the learner to touch the patient prior to performing a procedure, as it helps allay fears and provides a sense of connectedness. It may sound silly, but in a day and age of communicating largely via text messaging with minimal verbal and eye contact, there are likely some days when learners might never touch another person as they "practice" nursing. Does your facility follow a nursing philosophy? Then consider stating a few of the concepts as a piece of the education. An example is Watson's Caring Theory, which notes, "The dynamic of transpersonal caring (healing) within a caring moment is manifest in a field of consciousness" (Watson Caring Science Institute, 2015). Katharine Kolcaba's Comfort Theory (1991) goes a step further and provides the practicing nurse with a taxonomic structure to guide specifics on how to care (for example, comforting interventions).

Upon reviewing the list of learning paradigms, you will realize that the profession of nursing's own metaparadigm of nursing, environment, person, and health has roots in all of the learning paradigms! Thus the educator who is committed to ensuring that aspects of the nursing metaparadigm are incorporated into the design/development of learning activities is providing the nurse learner with a consistent framework (like the one shown in Figure 3.1) from which to make decisions of care.

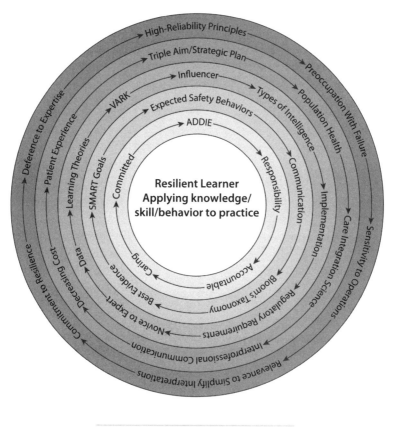

FIGURE 3.1

Metaparadigm of Nursing As Implemented by the Educator

Theories and Applications

Learning theories are information/proposals put forth to explain changes in behavior produced by practice, as opposed to other factors (Kimble, 2015). There are a few approaches to grouping theories together (based on a paradigm, worldview, or perspective) that serve as a starting point for our discussion. These broad categories of learning theories include:

- **Behaviorism.** A worldview that learners respond to external stimuli; in healthcare it is the ability of the healthcare giver to be aware of the effect the treatments are having on the patient/family.

- **Cognitivism.** The theory that moral judgments are statements of fact and can therefore be classed as true or false. In healthcare, it is the ability of the learner to apply critical thinking skills to the individual patient. Can the learner follow an algorithm or determine when to deviate?

- **Constructivism.** A philosophy of learning founded on the premise that, by reflecting on their experiences, individuals construct their own understanding of the world. In healthcare, the educator uses the Socratic method of questioning to assist the learners to base their care on their own previous experiences. For example, a learner who performs a skill in a simulation lab has most likely absorbed the procedural steps. When the skill is then performed in the clinical setting, the educator has the opportunity to guide the learner in developing a deeper understanding of the differences between what happens in the simulation lab vs. the real-world setting.

- **Humanism.** An outlook or system of thought that attaches prime importance to human rather than divine or supernatural matters. Humanist beliefs stress the potential value and goodness of human beings, emphasize common human needs, and seek solely rational ways of solving human problems. In healthcare, it is why compassion is a critical component in caring for the patient.

- **21st century skills.** Necessary for learners to be successful, such as digital and media literacy; for those in healthcare, this means knowledge of health literacy to help patients in understanding how to care for themselves.

We provide individual theories within several of these groupings in Table 3.2. The theories are provided as examples with corresponding considerations for the nursing professional development educator.

TABLE 3.2 _LEARNING THEORIES AND CONSIDERATIONS_

BEHAVIORIST THEORIES: A WORLDVIEW THAT LEARNERS RESPOND TO EXTERNAL STIMULI.	
Classical conditioning (Pavlov)	Nurse learners who have practiced in the same fashion for many years may need more skill practice than a new graduate nurse when a practice change is made.
	Educators should use simulation or train the trainer and include observation in the clinical setting to ensure the skill is being properly executed.
Operant conditioning (Skinner)	Nurse learners need positive reinforcement for continually performing best practice.
	Educators should use data and work with the manager to provide routine feedback (as opposed to during an annual performance evaluation only).
Social learning theory (Bandura)	Nurse learners acquire knowledge from each other via observation, imitation, and so on.
	Educators should focus on preparing preceptors for new graduate nurses as well as ensuring expert nurses are acting as champions for evidence-based practice (EBP).
COGNITIVIST THEORY: THE THEORY THAT MORAL JUDGMENTS ARE STATEMENTS OF FACT AND CAN THEREFORE BE CLASSED AS TRUE OR FALSE.	
Attribution theory (Weiner)	Nurse learners: Why do they do what they do?
	Educators should provide rationale for why the education must be completed and applied to practice.
Situated Learning (Lave)	Nurse learners have a responsibility to role model the caring aspects and best practice to students who can be considered apprentices.
	Educators can ensure the nurse learners are shown how to socialize students into the profession.

DESCRIPTIVE/META THEORY: DESCRIPTIVE/META THEORIES STATE HOW LEARNING OCCURS AND DEVISE MODELS THAT CAN BE USED TO EXPLAIN AND PREDICT LEARNING RESULTS.	
Bloom's taxonomy (Knowledge, Comprehension, Application, Analysis, Synthesis, and Evaluation)	Nurse learners who are aware of Bloom's taxonomy are able to understand how their level of nursing practice should advance over time, beginning as a novice new graduate and ending as an expert nurse capable of synthesizing and evaluating patient data.
	Educators should determine which level the education is targeted to and use the Socratic method as a means of ensuring the nurse learner succeeds (see the special feature that follows this table).

IDENTITY THEORY: IDENTITY THEORY IS A FAMILY OF VIEWS ON THE RELATIONSHIP BETWEEN MIND AND BODY.

Erikson's stages of development	Erikson's stages focus on the identity and psychosocial development of the individual, and the stages are easily transferable to interactions with nurse learners and patients/families.
	Educators should work to develop a *trusting* relationship with the nurse learners and lay the groundwork for a learner who can *self-actualize* his or her own lifelong learning.

MOTIVATIONAL/HUMANISTIC THEORIES: MOTIVATIONAL/HUMANISTIC THEORIES FOCUS ON THE LEARNER'S (SELF) MOTIVATION FOR LEARNING, NOT THE BEHAVIORS EXPECTED AS A RESULT OF THE LEARNING.

Emotional intelligence (Goleman)	Nurse learners who are aware of their emotional intelligence can use it to assist colleagues in reinforcing learning as part of teamwork.
	Educators should work to maintain self-awareness of their own emotional intelligence in order to better understand how to empathize with and motivate the nurse learners. The amount of education required of nurse learners in order to remain competent in their knowledge/skill/behavior for their specific population and role often means the educator considers including the "why" of responsibility and accountability for the learning.

continues

TABLE 3.2 *(CONTINUED)*

Experiential learning (Kolb)	Nurse learners benefit from education based upon Kolb's theory because it takes into consideration the need to experience learning in the work environment, such as a skills lab or simulation.
	Educators consider the cycle of experience, perception, cognition, and behavior while designing and developing the education. For example, what responsibility will the competent nurse learner have for informing the work of the new graduate nurse?
Maslow's hierarchy of needs (Maslow)	Nurse learners often struggle in their nursing practice (and healthcare in general) with self-actualization or self-fulfillment level. It could be of a personal nature that interferes with their practice, or the system the learner works in could be healthier.
	Educators working with the learner who has a desire for personal growth have a much easier time with helping the learner understand the need for education and subsequent practice change. Yet if the nurse learner is working in an unhealthy environment (similar to the Safety stage in this theory) or has not been socialized properly to the profession/facility (similar to Belongingness in this theory), the educator must work even more closely with the leadership to ensure all aspects of the nurse learner's struggles are under review.
SOCIAL DESIGN THEORIES: SOCIAL DESIGN THEORIES ARE DESCRIBED AS PREDICTING CERTAIN INTERGROUP BEHAVIORS ON THE BASIS OF PERCEIVED GROUP STATUS DIFFERENCES, THE PERCEIVED LEGITIMACY AND STABILITY OF THOSE STATUS DIFFERENCES, AND THE PERCEIVED ABILITY TO MOVE FROM ONE GROUP TO ANOTHER.	
ADDIE (Analyze, Design, Develop, Implement, Evaluate)	Nurse learners benefit from education developed based upon this method of instructional design simply because it is quite similar to the nursing process itself.
	Educators using the ADDIE model have a standardized approach that ensures a holistic approach to meeting the needs of the learner.

ARCS (Keller)	Nurse learners who receive education containing attention, relevance, confidence, and satisfaction (ARCS) are likely to be motivated to learn.
	Educators can ensure the inclusion of ARCS components in their education by including required demonstrations of skills to instill learner confidence. Providing rationale for why the education is needed helps the learners understand the relevance to their practice.
Multi-Modality (Kress)	Nurse learners communicate in a variety of ways with generations/ levels of other learners.
	Educators should take into account the various learning styles of the nurse learners and consider offering education using a variety of modalities.

MISCELLANEOUS THEORIES

Multiple intelligences theory (Gardner)—includes Naturalistic, Musical, Logical-Mathematical, Existential, Interpersonal, Bodily-Kinesthetic, Linguistic, Intra-personal, and Spatial intelligences	Nurse learners displaying certain types of intelligence may have the potential to take a larger role in the implementation portion of a continuing education (CE) activity. For example, should the learner who is "nature smart" and "bodily smart" act as the learner who pilots a learning activity? Should the learner who is "people smart" be part of the implementation/ evaluation portion of the plan?
	Educators can use multiple intelligence theory as a means of enhancing the implementation portion of the education plan by incorporating several of the intelligence types that will support different learning styles.

NOTE

For more information on learning theories, visit Richard Culatta's website on instructional design: http://www.instructionaldesign.org/theories. Culatta includes links to summaries, applications, examples, and principles of each of the learning theories described in Table 3.2; he also includes other popular learning theories.

SOCRATIC QUESTIONS TO ASK RELATED TO BLOOM'S TAXONOMY

If the nurse learner is gaining new knowledge, the Socratic questions should be at the comprehension level. Verbs for comprehension questions include compare, contrast, demonstrate, interpret, explain, extend, illustrate, infer, outline, relate, rephrase, translate, summarize, show, and classify. Sample questions could include "Could you explain what is happening…?" "How would you illustrate…?" "What might you infer from…?" and "Can you rephrase…?"

If the focus of the learning activity is on learning a new procedure, the Socratic questions should be at the application level: "What other way would you plan to…?" and "What would result if…?"

Learning Concepts

A *learning concept* is any idea or thought that the educator uses to facilitate learning. The professional development specialist uses any number of the following learning concepts (Culatta, 2013a) as a means of integrating content into the design of an educational program or learning activity:

- Anxiety
- Arousal
- Attention
- Attitudes
- Cognitive styles
- Creativity
- Grit and persistence
- Imagery
- Learning strategies
- Mastery
- Memory
- Mental models
- Metacognition
- Motivation
- Productions
- Reinforcement
- Schema
- Sequencing of instruction
- Taxonomies

For example, patient and employee safety depend on a shared mental model. A *mental model* is the nurse learner's perception of the clinical picture of the patient. It is the responsibility of the nurse learner to "share" that perception in order to create a clearer picture of what is happening with the patient and family. Having a shared mental model is one way all of the healthcare disciplines will contribute to the health of one patient, leading to change for a particular population as a whole. Acute Care, for example, uses the acronym SBARR (Situation, Background, Assessment, Recommendation, and Response) to standardize communication. As SBARR becomes the standard of communication across the continuum of care for all disciplines, the staff educator has the opportunity to drive the change by incorporating an SBARR example as education is designed. Are your preceptors taught to use SBARR to share information on how the new nurse learner is progressing? Remember the power of habit!

Other learning concepts the educator may choose to standardize for the nurse learners is the development of a taxonomy, and building the use of the Socratic method into the design of education so the learner thinks about his or her thinking (metacognition). As you design the education, consider adding reflective questions, such as how/when/where will the nurse learner apply the new knowledge or skill behavior into his or her practice? The use of taxonomy will support the educators who desire to build a curriculum for each of the various levels of the different roles for which they are responsible. Designing education activities or courses to fit into a curriculum and incorporating learning concepts will help the learners get to a shared mental model.

Learning Domains

A *domain* can be considered an area of focus, or a collection that is owned. In nursing, a common domain is professional relationships, and within that are specifics such as building a therapeutic relationship or knowledge of professional behaviors. Historically, professional development specialists have focused on the three domains of learning described in Table 3.3.

TABLE 3.3 *THREE DOMAINS OF LEARNING*

LEARNING DOMAIN	DESCRIPTION
Affective domain	Focuses on the emotions, feelings, beliefs, and values of an individual
Cognitive domain	Includes knowledge-based information pertaining to remembering, reasoning, and prioritizing (among other cognitive processes)
Psychomotor domain	Related to the hands-on skills or tangible aspects of knowledge

Although it's important for staff educators to understand these primary domains of learning, these aren't the only domains. Staff educators will find that it's important to consider some additional learning domains (Culatta, 2013b) when designing education:

- Computers
- Decision making
- Language
- Management
- Medicine
- Perception
- Problem solving
- Procedures
- Reading
- Reasoning
- Sensory-motor
- Troubleshooting

For example, the medicine domain is particularly noteworthy. Or consider the information on the reading domain, which provides the rationale for why slide presentations focus on bullet points. The domains of problem solving, reason, perception, and decision making are critical for educators to integrate into the design/development of education for the nurse learner.

> **NOTE**
>
> *Again, we recommend you check out Richard Culatta's website (http://www.instructionaldesign.org/domains/index.html) and review the additional learning domains that relate directly to the nurse learners' capacity to perform their duties. Upon review, the staff educator will note how the additional domains are directly related to specific learning theories. This connection hopefully helps illustrate the importance of understanding and using theories and models to frame one's work.*

Implications for Design

For the novice staff educator, simply reviewing a few of the education paradigms, theories, concepts, and domains will provide you with the beginnings of developing your own model. For the expert educator, the responsibility is to share your model with other educators. How wonderful would it be for nursing educators to lead the change toward population health from an educational perspective! Consider, for example, what might happen if educators started using a standardized model for educating the nurse learner and professionals from other disciplines on expectations for care along the continuum by choosing a topic such as health literacy to ensure that no patient is left behind.

As the educator uses the knowledge of theories to design the learning activity, the following design questions are asked:

- What did the needs assessment from the Analysis phase reveal? Is the gap in knowledge a skill or a behavior—or a combination of these components?

- Who/what are the internal and external resources? If you are the sole educator who performs all aspects of the ADDIE model, you may choose to see what uncopyrighted content is available online and then customize it to your specific facility. You could also start with a SlideShare presentation (http://www.slideshare.net), making sure to give credit to the original author, and then modify it to meet your nurse learner's needs.

- What is the available workplace support? What are the options for how to complete the learning activity? For example, as the sole educator, can you work with leadership to obtain a certain amount of the expert RNs' time to teach and observe the new skill or equipment?

- What about developing your own YouTube channel specific to your organization as a means of catching up learners who have been on leave, or as review for when annual skill check-offs are due?

- Are there constraints that exist related to location, budget, and technology expertise?

- Who are the subject matter experts that you can leverage to develop the content appropriate to meet the objectives?

- Have the outcomes for the nurse learner to be successful been identified? What are the knowledge, skills, and behaviors the learners should acquire as a result of the learning activity?

After the design questions have been answered, according to Dalto, "research demonstrates that you can use better training visuals to dramatically increase your learner's comprehension, retention, and transfer of behaviors to the workplace—and that's especially true for 'novice' learners who are new to a particular content area" (2014). You'll want to keep considering this as you begin to transition from the Design to Development of the learning activity.

Design Techniques That Enhance Training Materials

The use of visuals in training materials provides several benefits (like those listed in the preceding section) for learners. Staff educators should consider using the following graphic design techniques, which are drawn from Connie Malamed's book *Visual Language for Designers* (2014). (Malamed also has a blog, the eLearning Coach [http:// theelearningcoach.com], which educators should add to their Current Awareness list.)

> **NOTE**
>
> *"Current awareness" is a library of science term. It is the process by which the educator can set up a system where the information on specific topics comes to you versus you searching for information. We highly recommend a search of "setting up a system for current awareness" and setting up a system that will send alerts to your email, Twitter, or RSS feed service. For example, for the educator who is responsible for orientation of newly hired nurses, information from journals, libraries, and so on can all be sent to the educator who can access the RSS feed at any time or have the topic information go to a specific email folder set up to receive.*

- **Organize visuals so the learner will quickly and easily perceive the important elements.** Use features that pop out, different textures to draw attention, and group items within the visual.

- **Direct the learner's attention to the most important elements.** Position elements within the visual, emphasize elements, make use of movement (or the appearance of movement), direct the eyes of the viewer, and provide visual cues.

- **Use simplified visuals, as they are easier to process mentally.** Reduce visual noise, use silhouetted figures, make use of icons, incorporate line art, and let a single item represent larger numbers of the same item.

- **Make abstract or obscure concepts easier to understand by presenting the big-picture view.** Create easy-to-understand visualizations of data or other forms of information, use maps, and design visuals that include time as an element.

- **Make complex, complicated information easier to understand.** Present information visually in segments and/or sequences, use special views the human eye can't normally see, and use the structure of a graphic to help reinforce the graphic's intended meaning.

- **Use emotions, storytelling, surprise, and humor to increase attention and learning.** Add emotional elements to visuals, use visual storytelling techniques, create visual metaphors, and incorporate unexpected and/or humorous elements.

Let's look at an example using several of the techniques noted to help the nurse learner associate a new practice requirement with knowledge learned in school and used in daily practice. The practicing nurse automatically questions if the proper medication is being administered by using the 9 Rights of Medication Administration (yes, originally there were 5, then 7, and now 9). Recently, the International Organization for Standardization (ISO) published guidelines for ensuring tubing connections. The guidelines are identified in The Joint Commission Sentinel Alert 53 (2014) as "unrelated connectors fitting together well, provider inattention, poor lighting and other environmental factors, putting too many unrelated tubes in close proximity and not double-checking patients' tubes." Instead of sending out or posting the list, the educator creates the Six Rights to Connect outlined in the following steps. In doing so, the educator has used a format the learner is familiar with, drawn the learner's attention to the most important elements of the process, and made it easier to understand:

1. Why do I need this connection?

2. Did I follow the connection from the source to the patient?

3. Did I need to force the connection?

4. Is the fluid going into the right body system (IV to vein, NG to GI, and so on)?

5. How many adaptors do I need to make the connection? If more than one, get an independent verification.

6. If I find more than one connection or potential misconnection, I use STAR. (STAR is the safety acronym for Stop, Think, Act, and Review.)

Tips for Avoiding Visuals That Detract From Learning

Although we typically recommend training visuals when designing and developing a learning activity, there are several cases in which adding visuals might decrease the effectiveness of the training:

- **Adding visuals for purely decorative purposes.** Avoid using completely unrelated visuals simply for the sake of including artwork. For example, don't add a clip art picture of a smiling sun in the corner of a slide presentation about safety behaviors.

- **Adding marginally related visuals that do not directly support the learning objectives.** Restrain yourself from including visuals that are somewhat related but are included only because they seem "interesting." For example, if your training materials are designed to teach proper blood administration techniques, resist adding an image of a zombie from *The Walking Dead*. This artwork certainly isn't humorous, helpful, or appropriate, only distracting.

- **Adding so many images that the learner's working memory is overloaded, or adding visuals that otherwise detract from the learning experience.** For *initial* education activities in nursing, training materials should note only the *need* to know—not the *nice* to know. Note, however, that with initial education the educator and the subject matter expert often disagree. The subject matter experts want to give the learner ALL the knowledge they have, forgetting it may have taken them countless years to reach their current practice level. To prevent this overload from happening, the educator develops a set of simple questions that can be given to any subject matter expert:

- What is the rationale for the education (such as strategic initiative, safety-related, regulatory requirement, interprofessional request, new procedure or equipment)?

- What are the expected learner outcomes in relation to the goal of the education from your perspective (change in knowledge/skill/behavior/combination)?

- What is the proposed timeframe for the education?

- What data are available to support the evaluation?

- What do you see as the role of the subject matter expert?

- What is the expected documentation of the nurse learner?

After these questions have been answered, the educator can begin to design, develop, and, more important, determine whether this education can be *integrated* into other proposed education. Why? Because the nurse learner often views each learning activity as separate from the other. This is why the educator incorporates appropriate aspects of the care continuum, such as documentation, patient education, and communication across disciplines, as reminders to the learner that each new learning activity must be incorporated into practice.

- **Simple materials should be created for both of the brain's processing systems.** Educators must recognize the importance of using both visual and auditory means of education because the mind must filter, select, organize, and integrate the presented information. Recall and recognition are enhanced by using both visual and verbal forms. (See dual coding theory and multimedia theory for additional information.) Thus the educator will want to add voice-over commentary to a slide presentation when warranted, or insert sound into a video. For more information, search online for "ways to make learning materials."

Implications for Development

After the educator has thought about the design of the education, the following points should be reviewed during the development phase:

- What is the best content delivery system for the education? eLearning, classroom, webinar, skill blitz, case study, lecture, group discussion, or some combination? This is a key point where the staff educator considers the learning theories, the nurse learners' characteristics, and the desired outcomes.

- What method of evaluation will be used? (See Chapter 5, "Evaluating an Individual's Growth," and Chapter 6, "Evaluating an Educational Program's Performance," for some ideas.) And when is the learner responsible for implementing the new knowledge/skill/behavior?

- Evaluation is an area where the educator has the opportunity to support a just culture within patient safety. Take the opportunity to remind the learner of the facility's values and how those relate to the learning activity. Discuss the expectations of when the education is to be applied in practice (and consequences for not applying the learnings to practice). Inform the learner of steps to take if there is a system issue, and who the resources are for follow-up.

- Create a checklist or Gantt chart for each phase of the program. Be sure to include corresponding timelines and note who is responsible for each step of the checklist. Send to all involved to help everyone adhere to the timelines and send periodic emails to check on progress.

An Example of the Design and Development Process

Instead of speaking only in generalizations, let's consider some realistic examples of how to incorporate design and development principles into educational activities. This section begins with a description of a "core" competency that focuses on essential information for all clinicians. It then covers "ongoing" competency, which focuses on new knowledge, skills, and behaviors that surface intermittently.

Core Competency

In 2012, Medicare began penalizing hospitals that have high readmission rates. Nationally, about 18% of all patients discharged to nursing homes are readmitted within 30 days. According to an article by Butcher (2015), to make a difference in readmission rates, there needed to be transformation in the four areas noted here:

1. **Selection of the right "first setting" for the patient being discharged from the hospital.** Discharge planning begins on the day of admission. What is the responsibility of the individual nurse in his or her work setting for where the patient currently is along the continuum of care? How does the educator teach the nurse learner to be proactive in what the patient will need during the next phase of his or her healthcare journey? Certainly one method is by supporting the next area: standardization.

2. **Standardization across the continuum of care.** Standardization is critical to nursing moving forward as a profession. It is the opportunity for the educator who works for a large system that encompasses primary care, clinics, acute care, home care, skilled nursing facilities, and so on to work with colleagues to standardize portions of education for the nurse learner so both the patients/families as well as staff know the expectations.

3. **Longitudinal care planning.** Ah, yes, care plans—the hallmark of nursing care. The staff educator has the opportunity to reinforce the role each nurse learner plays along the continuum. How novel if the educator and colleagues taught the nurse learners what comes before versus what comes after they provide care. This might help nurses regain ownership of their practice and their role as coordinator of patient care.

4. **The use of nurse care navigators to help patients transition successfully from one care setting to another.** As the leadership plans and activates new roles such as nurse navigator to assist with movement along the continuum of care and toward population health, what does the nurse learner need to know about the new roles to be supportive? Here is where the educator has the opportunity to assist. For example, in designing and developing a learning activity related to patient education, the educator could include the importance of why those working as nurse navigators may need to be apprised of the status of the patient education via the electronic health record.

Please consider what your facility has already implemented to prevent readmissions, and ask whether or not you as the educator took the opportunity or knew of the opportunity to educate the nurse learners to support the efforts. The additional thoughts noted below each of the preceding points are based upon the premise that preventing readmissions could be considered a core competency across the care continuum. Think of the impact on individual patient outcomes as well as the Triple Aim if professional development specialists used a standardized process across the care continuum.

Ongoing Competency

How much time does the educator waste by glossing over things, rushing through things, or being distracted while trying to impart new learning as part of an ongoing competency? How does the educator decide if the learner needs to review all previous content? It can sometimes be wasteful (and, dare we say, lazy) to have all learners repeat the same content on an annual basis. Consider performing routine mini-analyses like the following:

- A knowledge/skill check-up front

- A review of incident report data or any other data collected related to the planned education

- A check-in with the subject matter expert to determine whether there is new evidence that needs to be incorporated

- A few observations to determine the quality of the current practice (that is, might there be a specific area that has been "forgotten" by most learners?)

Education related to ongoing competencies should be designed and developed to take the learner to the next level. The competency itself should have become standardized practice, and the annual review can be designed to assist the learners to take their practice to the next level as evidenced by being a master at skills as well as understanding their own motivation and need for feedback.

For example, would you consider recognizing the signs and symptoms of sepsis as an ongoing competency? As it is the nurse learner who essentially prevents the patient from becoming septic, the necessary knowledge should be incorporated as part of any related education. All patients have the potential to show a decline in vital signs, change in cap refill, or change in mental status (often the first sign in the elderly), and the first 12 hours after noticing a decline in status are critical. For example, the primary focus of a learning activity might be to learn how to care for the patient with an indwelling urinary (Foley) catheter. The planned content could simply have been the rationale for insertion, proper technique for insertion, and maintenance/removal of the catheter. Yet shouldn't the signs/symptoms of infection be noted as part of the education? Because much of care is based upon task, it's the RN as the coordinator of care who must have all the pieces of the puzzle to assist in critical thinking.

Technology Considerations During Design and Development

We'll spend a bit more time in Chapter 8, "Putting Technology to Work for You," discussing technology, but during the Design and Development phase, you'll at least want to consider the following:

- Will the education be entered into the learning management system?

- Will the education be for both newly hired and experienced learners? If so, will it need to be posted in two different areas?

- Will technology be able to support the need for review when the knowledge/skill/behavior is actually needed?

- How is the electronic health record supporting the education and evaluation of the implementation?

- How does technology impact communication related to the education? What happens to the work of the educator when the systems are not integrated?

Both the educator and the learner must always take into account the impact the use of technology has on daily practice. From a learning perspective, technology can help to reinforce education by having reminders built into the electronic medical record. The reminders could automatically activate for the first 30 days of the practice change and then be deleted. Eventually this should be able to happen for the individual learner, so that specific reminders can be turned on for every new hire. In terms of tracking education via the learning management system, technology should assist the educator in providing the individual learner with a curriculum based upon the learner's goals, the patient population the learner is working with, the organization's core values, and the nursing profession's standards of care. Doing so would narrow the gap of most needs assessments related to the learners as well as meet the Triple Aim. Designing and developing content is much more effective when there is a supportive technological framework.

Conclusion

By designing and developing the learning activity, the professional development specialist is using knowledge/skill/behaviors of the practice of education. Owning the practice of education influences how the nurse learner owns the practice of nursing. The staff educator stays abreast of the changes in healthcare that will affect the specific nurse learners with whom he or she works by setting up Current Awareness. The educator uses Current Awareness to learn about the latest evidence in learning theories, as well as technology and methods of designing/developing education in a variety of formats. The educator remembers the mantra of "need to know versus nice to know," the importance of always including resources for the learner, and the desire to assist the learner with how to integrate new knowledge/skill/behavior into his/her current practice. The staff educator will want to become knowledgeable about implementation science and consider its usefulness after the Analysis, Design, Develop portions of the ADDIE model are complete. Just as the educator requests the learner be forward-thinking on behalf of the patient, the educator needs to be forward-thinking on behalf of the learner by using methods to promote the integration of research findings and evidence into the practice of education.

Questions for Reflection/Discussion

1. Why should the educator use a learning theory? How does it help develop and design the learning activity?

2. What are questions the educator should ask about the effect technology has on the Develop and Design portions of the ADDIE model?

3. When developing and designing education around a new piece of equipment, what domains of learning does the educator take into account in developing and designing the education?

KEY TAKEAWAYS

- *The educator leverages beneficial learning theories and models, recognizes organizational resources and limitations, and continues to engage key stakeholders when designing and developing educational activities.*

- *The educator is aware of the nursing metaparadigm (person, health, nursing, environment), and ensures that the design and development of content can be traced back to at least one of the components.*

- *The educator considers the current practice and competency of the learner in designing and developing educational activities.*

Resources

Benner, P., Kyriakidis, P., & Stannard, D. (2011). *Clinical wisdom and interventions in acute and clinical care* (2nd ed.). New York, NY: Springer.

Culatta, R. (2013). Learning theories. Retrieved from http://www.instructionaldesign.org/theories

Duhigg, C. (2014). *The power of habit: Why we do what we do in life and business*. New York, NY: Random House.

References

Butcher, L. (2015). Why nursing home quality matters to hospitals. *Trustee*. Retrieved from http://www.trusteemag.com/display/TRU-news-article.dhtml?dcrPath=/templatedata/HF_Common/NewsArticle/data/TRU/Magazine/2015/Mar/COV_SNFquality_nursing_homes&utm_source=insidetru&utm_medium=email&utm_campaign=TRU

Campinha-Bacote, J. (2002). The process of cultural competence in the delivery of healthcare services: A model of care. *Journal of Transcultural Nursing, 13*(3), 181–184. doi: 10.1177/10459602013003003

Culatta, R. (2013a). Learning concepts. Retrieved from http://www.instructionaldesign.org/concepts/index.html

Culatta, R. (2013b). Learning domains. Retrieved from http://www.instructionaldesign.org/domains/index.html

Dalto, J. (2014). How to design great training materials: 25 techniques for better training visuals. Retrieved from http://blog.convergencetraining.com/how-to-design-great-training-materials

Institute for Healthcare Improvement. (2015). IHI Triple Aim initiative. Retrieved from http://www.ihi.org/engage/initiatives/TripleAim/Pages/default.aspx

Institute of Medicine. (2010). *The future of nursing: Leading change, advancing health*. Washington, DC: National Academies Press. Retrieved from http://www.iom.edu/Reports/2010/The-Future-of-Nursing-Leading-Change-Advancing-Health.aspx

The Joint Commission. (2014). Managing risk during transition to new ISO tubing connector standards. *Sentinel Alert,* (53). Retrieved from http://www.jointcommission.org/assets/1/6/SEA_53_Connectors_8_19_14_final.pdf

Kimble, G. (2015). Learning theory. In *Encyclopaedia Britannica.* Retrieved from http://www.britannica.com/EBchecked/topic/334034/learning-theory

Kolcaba, K. Y. (1991). A taxonomic structure for the concept comfort. *Journal of Nursing Scholarship*, *23*(4), 237–240. Retrieved from http://thecomfortline.com/files/pdfs/1991%20-%20Taxonomic%20Structure%20of%20Comfort%20Theory.pdf

Malamed, C. (2014). The eLearning Coach. Retrieved from http://theelearningcoach.com/

paradigm. (2015). In *Oxforddictionaries.com.* Retrieved from http://www.oxforddictionaries.com/us/definition/american_english/paradigm

Watson Caring Science Institute. (2015). Caring science theory & research. Retrieved from http://watsoncaringscience.org/about-us/caring-science-definitions-processes-theory

CHAPTER 4

Implementing Professional Development Activities

Introduction

If you're reading this book's chapters in order, you might be wondering how you will begin to apply all of these high-level concepts into the real work of the professional development specialist. Well, if that's your thought, then this chapter, which covers the Implementation step of the ADDIE model, is for you! We'll be providing you with the *how* by looking at the *who, what, when, where,* and *why* of professional development activities, though not necessarily in the order listed here. Using these five W's of learning activity and educational program development within the ADDIE model is the perfect formula to use for successful education planning.

Why Is the Activity Necessary?

Nurses today face many knowledge gaps in providing safe and efficient patient care. With higher patient acuities, more complex chronic care populations, and new technology surfacing every day, one way to help nurses adapt seamlessly to new practices is to provide thoughtfully planned out education. This education needs to be supported with data and examples of how change can improve practice, patient outcomes, and patient safety.

Hopefully we have convinced you that using the ADDIE model as a guide for developing educational activities is a must. After examining the results (likely from multiple sources) in the Analysis phase, learning activities are designed and developed. The American Nurses Credentialing Center states that identifying learning needs through data collection is crucial to the preplanning of any learning activity (ANCC, 2014). The following steps demonstrate how the ANCC organizes this pre-implementation work:

1. Review available data sources (qualitative and quantitative) that can assist in preparing the needs assessment.

2. Conduct a needs assessment to identify the gap or verify a known gap in knowledge, skill, or attitude (behavior).

3. Design and develop the learning activity based upon the results of the needs assessment.

Performing these steps consistently will not only lay a solid foundation for a successful learning activity, but also prepare you to share the rationale for the activity with learners and other stakeholders.

When a knowledge gap has been identified (see Chapter 2), staff educators must be sure to incorporate the rationale behind the need for education into the learning activity itself. Adult learners link knowledge with past experiences and are problem centered. As a result, in order for learners to "buy into" or integrate new knowledge into current practice, they must find value in the identified knowledge gap. By showing the data used to help identify the gap as part of the learning activity, the educator is providing the learners with rationale for why content was designed and developed to close the gap. The educator desires that the learner values the education in order to apply the new knowledge, skill, and attitude into daily practice. Ways to provide the rationale for education include:

1. Use the data to market the upcoming activity. Disseminate the pre-education data findings, and the goal for post-education findings.

2. Include pieces of data in the content itself.

3. Demonstrate how the data is connected with patient outcomes.

Sometimes, the rationale for requiring learners to complete a learning activity is as simple as including a one-sentence statement with the activity's announcement. For example, completing yearly Occupational Safety and Health Administration (OSHA) and Disaster Preparedness Review to meet The Joint Commission (TJC) requirements doesn't necessitate a lengthy rationale because this is a requirement to maintain compliance with a regulatory body. The rationale could be as simple as "Complete for OSHA/TJC yearly required education/review." Other times (especially if the activity is time-consuming or in other ways burdensome), you might need to describe the need to complete this activity as it relates to patient care. For example, if there is an issue on the unit with increased pressure ulcer rates, you could describe downward trends in a performance improvement monitor (like pressure ulcer prevention compliance) and how this affects patient outcomes.

DESCRIBING THE WHY OF A LEARNING ACTIVITY

Let's say you just asked learners to complete a newly developed learning activity for preventing pressure ulcers. In response, one of the experienced nurses in your area shows her resistance by making a comment like, "I have done at least a hundred education modules in my career on pressure ulcers, and I think I know how to do this by now." Although there are a couple options for dealing with this scenario (including an assessment of the staff member's attitude and the need to consider whether other work environment factors could be bothering this person), when it comes to explaining a rationale you could try the following statements:

- *If quality indicators had identified practice gaps—"If I could show you our pressure ulcer rates over the last few audits, you'll see we have had an increase in trends. We are trying several interventions, and we want to be certain that all of our staff members are aware of the current policies and procedures on these interventions. Will you help us with these efforts?"*

> • *If staff interviews had identified that several nurses were unfamiliar with the guidelines—"We checked in with staff members in our most recent staff meeting, and there seemed to be a high level of concern regarding everyone's comfort level with what is and isn't found in the prevention guidelines. Although it seemed like the greatest concern was among those who haven't been working in the unit a very long time, we weren't sure where to make a cut-off of who should and shouldn't complete the activity. If you feel pretty comfortable with the guidelines, would you be willing to help us out by serving as a unit resource for inexperienced staff members?"*

One external source that highlights the importance of many learning activities is within the Quality and Safety Education for Nurses (QSEN) competencies. As many new nurse learners will be familiar with (and the experienced learners can begin to understand from where the millennials are gathering their ideas in academia), QSEN and another more recent initiative, the Campaign for Action, highlight the need for transforming healthcare delivery.

To illustrate how this helps with understanding the *why* of a learning activity, let's say there is a need to provide a repeated learning activity for a documentation issue. Cronenwett et al. (2007) in *Nursing Outlook* is the basis for the work QSEN developed regarding the knowledge, skill, and attitudes the learner requires to document successfully. If you were to review the QSEN competency on informatics, for example, you would find *informatics* to be defined as using "information and technology to communicate, manage knowledge, mitigate error, and support decision making" (Cronenwett et al., 2007). The nursing professional would need to employ the following skills:

- Navigate the electronic medical record (EMR).
- Document and plan patient care in an EMR.
- Employ communication technologies to coordinate care for patients.
- Understand the EMR serves as the legal document of care provided.

For staff educators, reinforcing the knowledge nurse learners should already have is always an important piece of assisting them in integrating additional knowledge. For example, a learning activity is developed for a central venous catheter dressing change procedural guideline. By reinforcing each step of the dressing change procedure in the development of the learning activity, nurse learners can identify steps that they may have not been following during patient care and focus on incorporating these missed steps into their practice.

Check out Table 4.1 for a summary of the questions to consider for the first W—*why*.

TABLE 4.1   *ASKING THE* WHY *OF A LEARNING ACTIVITY*

COMPONENT	QUESTIONS TO ASK
Rationale	What is the reason for this learning activity? (Should relate directly to the Analysis phase [for example, practice gaps, staff concerns, regulatory requirements])
Promotion to Learners	How will you promote the activity to learners to gain their buy-in? (For example, one-sentence summary, full explanation, sharing full details of practice gaps)

NOTE

For your convenience, we combine each of the Ws in the worksheet shown on page 95.

Who Should Attend the Activity?

When planning a learning activity, staff educators need to develop the activity to accommodate the target audience, the *who*. The *target audience* is a group of staff members with an identified knowledge gap.

For example, if the learning activity is designed for direct patient care providers, *who* specifically is part of the target audience? Does it include RNs, LPNs, unlicensed assistive personnel (UAP), or all care providers, including the management team, ancillary staff, and advanced practice staff? If the education involves multiple disciplines, will a single learning activity meet each discipline's learning needs, or should different classes on the subject matter be tailored for each discipline? For example, education on the use of restraints may require tailored information for different disciplines. The RN's learning activity might require information on de-escalation techniques, provider order requirements, application of restraints, assessment and safety requirements when using restraints, evaluation of the effectiveness, when to safely remove the restraints, and required documentation. The UAP may only require de-escalation techniques, application and safety considerations, and when to call the RN. If, however, the UAP attends the RN learning activity, the UAP's key focus items would be lost in the higher-level details that an RN would require. If different audiences require different content (or even different delivery modes/styles), educators should separate the learning activities to meet these individual learning needs.

Establishing who should be present for a learning activity is also a consideration for a larger scale conference, such as a certification review course. The educator needs to decide whether the learning activity will be open to employees working at the institution only or be open to external customers, but first the educator must determine the number of internal staff desiring to attend the conference. Limiting attendance of the learning activity allows more opportunity for the institution's targeted audience to attend. However, if institutional needs are met and there is an outside interest in the content presented, it could be opened to outside customers if the speaker and facilities can accommodate additional learners.

The speaker or subject matter expert (SME) is the educator's next consideration when developing a learning activity. Is the bedside educator always the best option for presenting a learning activity? Not always, and that is OK. Many institutions have SMEs who are better options for facilitating a learning activity. If using an SME, the educator then manages the activity, facilitating what is needed for the speaker to make the learning activity successful. For example, if the use of high-fidelity simulation is needed in order to stimulate more critical thinking and problem solving, the educator would work with the SME to develop the activity, but the SME would actually run the simulation and the planned education.

IS THE STAFF EDUCATOR THE BEST FACILITATOR?

Many times, the staff educator designs and develops all of the education for a nursing unit. But is the staff educator always the right person? The unit-based educator might have several favorite topics in his or her wheelhouse of presentations, but, if resources and opportunity arise, it might be a better option to utilize SMEs within one's organization to develop the education.

Let's say your unit will now be pulling femoral sheaths on post-cardiac catheterization patients instead of the procedure being done by Cardiac Cath. Lab staff. The experts on pulling femoral sheaths (the current cath. lab nursing staff) should be the SMEs in developing the education on appropriate techniques, protocols, and post cath. complications. As a bonus to developing and providing the training for your staff members taking over the skill set, an additional result is developing improved communication and trust between units that will be closely working together in the future.

Another example of when to look outside may be when you are asked to develop an organization-wide education on a Healthy Work Environment inservice, and you would like to bring in an outside speaker. You might consider going to the American Association of Critical-Care Nurses (ACCN) Speakers Bureau (http://www.aacn.org/wd/hwe/content/speakers.content?lastmenu) to find a speaker on this topic. Another speaker bureau is Sigma Theta Tau International's Speakers Bureau (http://www.sttispeakersbureau.org).

Regardless of who does the actual teaching, it takes a small village to successfully deliver a learning activity. Many people and departments are needed to plan and implement an activity, which includes the following tasks:

- Contracting with a speaker and, if the speaker is coming from out of town, making travel and lodging arrangements

- Making arrangements for classroom assignment or conference hall

- Completing the continuing education (CE) application and coordinating procurement of required CE documents

- Printing CE evaluations and certificates

- Creating and distributing flyers that advertise the learning activity

- Registering participants

- Printing any materials to be distributed to learners

- Creating a registration/sign-in sheet and greeting participants

- Setting up catering (if food will be provided)

- Making arrangements for and setting up and assisting with audiovisual equipment

- Assisting with setting up equipment needed for the learning activity (for example, pumps, simulation materials, and so on)

- Assisting with any activities that will be completed during the learning activity

Table 4.2 summarizes considerations for the *who* of a learning activity.

TABLE 4.2 *ASKING THE* WHO *OF A LEARNING ACTIVITY*

COMPONENT	QUESTIONS TO ASK
Disciplines	Which disciplines will comprise the target audience? (For example, RNs, UAPs, physicians, social workers)
Internal versus External	Which units/departments will you invite? Will the activity be limited only to your organization?
Presenters	Who will be your presenter(s)/facilitator(s)?

When Will the Activity Take Place?

There never seems to be a perfect time—the *when*—for a learning activity, especially when planning an activity in which bedside nurses or other direct care providers from a 24-hour patient care unit will be required or heavily encouraged to attend. The staff educator must juggle times that work with the schedules of off-shift staff and the business needs of the nursing unit. Flexibility is the name of the game. For example, offering multiple classes on different days and at different times may encourage attendance, especially if the learning activity is required for all staff.

If learners work in an area that does not require 24/7 coverage, staff educators should consider working with the area's manager to designate a date and time for educational activities. Examples might include "every Wednesday morning before seeing any patients" or "the first Tuesday of each quarter."

Unfortunately, timing is not always in the hands of the educator. Does the knowledge gap require immediate intervention and need to be conducted *yesterday*? Or does the educator have time to plan the activity over a 6 to 9 month timeframe? Is the knowledge gap eligible for CE credits? These questions are items to consider when planning when a learning activity will take place. Using a timetable will assist the educator to keep on target with required tasks and ensure their completion prior to the time the activity takes place. In addition to the Gantt chart mentioned in Chapter 3, Figures 4.1 and 4.2 provide some examples on organizing a timeline for a learning activity.

Speakers also have an influence on when a learning activity will be conducted, especially if the SME is from outside your institution or from out of town. Most speakers will try to be flexible in their ability to present the learning activity, but be prepared for limitations. If using an SME from outside your institution, create a written agreement/contract with the SME after you've agreed upon date(s) and time(s) for the learning activity.

If introducing new equipment into your facility, ask whether the company has staff members dedicated to assisting with the rollout of the product and delivery of education to your staff members. If so, include in the purchase contract the availability of the company's education department to meet off-shift training sessions. For example, if planning education on a new infusion pump, off-shift class times would allow for evening and night-shift staff to attend the class during their working shifts. The company educators will be flexible if attendance can be assured. If the equipment company does not have such resources, you might consider having a few interested staff members attend more than one product demonstration and designate them as resources for other staff members (some facilities call these staff members "super users").

Marketing the Activity

After it has been determined when to offer the learning activity, you want to focus on marketing to allow staff members' adequate time to incorporate the class into their work-life schedules. Providing staff enough time in advance to work education into their planning schedule encourages improved attendance. If you work in an organization where learners' schedules are not fixed (for example, where schedules are made in blocks of 6-week periods), planning a learning activity during a current schedule cycle might be difficult for learners to alter their schedules to attend the activity. If the advertisement is 1 to 2 months ahead of the current schedule cycle, learners can incorporate and plan for the event. Attendance is greater when there is advanced planning and advertisement.

Date Due	Date Completed	Description
9–12 Months Out		
		Form the committee.
		Identify objectives of conference, goal, target audience.
		Complete a needs assessment.
		Create a budget.

Day of Conference		
		Arrive at least 1 hour prior to registration.
		Connect with venue liaison immediately.
		Post signage, if needed.
		Set up registration, if needed.
		Speaker introduction/room moderation.
		Treasurer present with checkbook to pay speakers, venue, other expenses. Note: Be sure to have all speakers complete and sign a W-9 Form (http://www.irs.gov/pub/irs-pdf/fw9.pdf) before paying them their fee.
		Keep a list of suggestions that arise during the event for future conference(s).
		Provide program evaluation to all attendees.
		Provide learning evaluation to all attendees (pre/post test).
		Hand out CNE certificates to all attendees.

FIGURE 4.1

Sample Timeline for Planning a Local Activity
Source: American Association of Critical-Care Nurses (2012).

CONFERENCE PLANNING TIMELINE

APPROX. 1 YEAR PRIOR TO EVENT
- Begin completing requests for continuing education (CE) credits with a CE planner.
- Once program is approved by CE planner, set up planning group meeting (determine meeting frequency).
- Select a site/venue for the event.
- Begin to determine budget and additional timelines.

APPROX. 9 MONTHS PRIOR TO EVENT
- Begin speaker selection/agenda development.
- Sign contracts for meeting space, hotel, social event, etc.
- Develop marketing plan and/or begin to collect mailing lists, listserv information, etc.
- Determine registration method (set up website, if available).

APPROX. 6 MONTHS PRIOR TO EVENT
- Continue planning team meetings.
- Mail "Save the Date" postcard to target audience.
- Finalize speaker(s) and agenda.
- Send out speaker packets with required materials and timelines.
- Draft brochure with conference objectives.
- Mail marketing information (flyers, brochures, quarterly calendar, etc.) after review by a CE planner.
- Discuss food menu options, if applicable.

60 DAYS PRIOR TO EVENT
- Submit all required CE activity information to the CE planner for review.
- Determine food menu.
- Follow up on any necessary speaker information.
- Assign planning team responsibilities for day of activity.

30 DAYS PRIOR TO EVENT
- Ensure CE documentation is accurate and complete.
- Create activity sign-in sheet and evaluation form (in collaboration with CE planner).
- Submit projected menu counts to caterer.

ACTUAL EVENT DATE
- Collect completed sign-in sheet and evaluation forms for each participant.

30 DAYS AFTER EVENT DATE
- Participant contact hour credit applied
- Activity closed

FIGURE 4.2

Sample Timeline for Planning a Large Conference
Source: Cincinnati Children's Hospital Medical Center (2014).

WHEN THE ACTIVITY NEEDS TO BE DONE ASAP

Unfortunately, there are times when planning a learning activity simply isn't possible (for example, a serious patient care error occurred, and the organization's staff requires immediate training). In these instances, staff educators must work with the manager and/or scheduling personnel to determine how to provide coverage for current patient care needs while assisting staff members in attending a learning activity. In some cases, the educator might need to cover a learner's patient assignment while the learner attends the activity. (Although this isn't ideal, it can have the unintended benefit of demonstrating to staff members that the educator values professional development and patient care and that these are not mutually exclusive activities.)

Some thought needs to be put into planning the advertisement of a learning activity. When creating a flyer or a brochure for the learning activity, include the following details:

- A clear description of the learning activity

- A description of the target audience, including required and optional attendees

- A brief explanation of the educational program, including associated learning objectives

- An agenda

- Information on whether contact hours are offered (if so, include a state board-approved CE statement)

- Any fees required of attendees

- A clear indication of registration deadlines

- The procedure for canceling registration

- Complete contact information

If the learning activity provides CE hours, then all of the preceding information is required in the flyer or brochure. If the educational program is more than one day in length, you should also include a complete multi-day agenda. If learners external to your organization will attend, it's beneficial to include information on travel, lodging, and recreational activities.

Setting Completion Deadlines for Learners

If learners can complete the learning activity in a self-paced or self-scheduled manner (for example, reviewing an educational poster or completing an online module), the staff educator should set due dates for learners. After the activity is available to learners, it might be unreasonable to expect all of them to complete the activity within just a few days. (For example, what if patient census or acuity unexpectedly increases, and the learners need to divert all attention to patient care?) However, if the activity must be completed before a significant practice or policy change, it might be necessary to enforce deadlines.

In some situations, especially if the learning activity does not require significant time or cognitive focus, the activity can be completed during an assigned shift where active patient care is not being provided. For example, you assign staff members to complete an online module for their yearly review of emergency preparedness for fires (frequently known as "Code Red"). This particular module will only take 15 minutes to complete and, in most cases, is a review of standard Code Red practices. Many staff members may have a reasonable amount of down time in which to complete the learning module. The educator should work in conjunction with the unit leader/manager to determine whether it's appropriate to complete learning activities while performing patient care. It can be a struggle to determine whether integrating learning activities is appropriate, and one might consider factors such as patient census/acuity, domain of learning, and time when making this decision.

Table 4.3 summarizes the *when* aspects of implementation.

TABLE 4.3 *ASKING THE* **WHEN** *OF A LEARNING ACTIVITY*

COMPONENT	QUESTIONS TO ASK
Importance	Do you have sufficient time to plan an ideal activity, or does the activity need to occur ASAP?
Learners' Schedules	Will all interested (or required) learners be able to attend the learning activity at a single point in time? If not, how many activities need to be held, and what variation in time should occur to accommodate all learners?
Timeline	What does a brief outline of your timeline (starting with what could be done *this week*) look like?
Facilitators	Who are your facilitators, and what are the constraints on their schedules?
Deadlines	By when must the learning activity be completed, and is this sufficient time for learners to complete the activity?

Where Will the Activity Take Place?

Where to have a learning activity largely depends on what type of education is to be conducted. Audio-visual (AV) services and how the room is organized are major components to consider when scheduling a location for a learning activity. Once the needs of the room are determined to conduct an education, the classroom can be reserved.

To determine the best venue for a learning activity, staff educators should consider the answers to the questions in Table 4.4.

TABLE 4.4   *ASKING THE* WHERE *OF A LEARNING ACTIVITY*

COMPONENT	QUESTIONS TO ASK
Location	Should education occur at the point of care or away from the nursing unit?
	Should the activity occur offsite?
	What type of AV equipment/support is available at the location?
	What type/how much equipment will need to be brought in?
Attendance	What is the anticipated number of attendees?
	Internal attendees only?
	External attendees?
Setup	What format (simulation, case scenarios, interactive activities, lecture, and so on) is used to conduct the activity?
	Do you need tables to support group discussion or group activities? Stations to conduct multiple skill checks?
	Is AV equipment needed for demonstration purposes? Will the activity be filmed for repeated use?
	What healthcare-related equipment is needed (for example, IV poles, dressing kits, and so on)?
	Are patient simulators needed?
	Do facilitators need a table?
	Do you need an area for posters or for equipment to display?
	Do you need tables for food or drink?
	Do you need a registration table?

COMPONENT	QUESTIONS TO ASK
Budget	Budget support and cost of conducting education at a hotel or conference center vs classroom or conference within the institution?
	If providing food/beverages, does the location support this function provided by facility?
	Costs of providing/supporting AV equipment at a hotel/ conference center vs classroom or conference center within the institution?

What Is the Budget and What Format Is Best?

When it comes to the *what* component of the Ws, staff educators must consider two different "what" questions. The first involves budget (what are the expenses?), and the second involves format (what setup will work best?). We discuss budget first, because budget often has a significant impact on the format used.

Making a Budget Plan

The budget—what expenses will be incurred—plays a huge role in the development of an educational program. The expenses (and revenue earned) from an individual activity can greatly impact the larger educational program's budget. Staff educators have many cost considerations when planning a budget:

- Honorarium for speakers
- Travel, lodging, and dining expenses for out-of-town speakers
- Program materials and supplies (handouts, folders, jump drives, and so on)
- Printing of posters and graphics
- AV rental or other equipment rental costs
- Catering expenses
- Office supplies (name tags, pens, pencils, paper clips, staplers, receipts)

- Cost of paying staff to attend required learning activities (non-clinical time) and any overtime costs to cover patient care on the nursing unit

- Sponsors or vendors providing financial support for the educational program

In addition to considering the items in the preceding list, also take into account whether staff or unit budgets will be required to pay for the educational opportunity. If so, what will that fee cover and how much will the fee be?

If an activity is planned early enough, the staff educator can determine approximate expenses for the above items. The staff educator can then work with the manager to incorporate expenses for learning activities in the yearly budget. Worksheet 4.1 shows a budget template that you can modify to meet your needs.

Expenses	Item	Cost/Unit	Number of Units	Amount Budgeted	Actual Expense
	Marketing: Flyers	$0.50	500	$250	$264.30
	Marketing: Mailing List Purchase	$750	1	$750	$750.00
	Salary: Planning Staff	$35/hr.	40	$1,400	$1,400.00
	Room Rental	$250	1	$250	$250.00
	Speaker: Honorarium	$500	1	$500	$500.00
	Speaker: Travel	$600	1	$600	$575.90
	Catering	$25	150	$3,750	$3,150.00
	Printing Costs	$5	150	$750	$636.25
			Total Expenses = $8,250.00		$7,526.45
Revenues	Registration	$90	125	$11,250	$10,350
	Exhibitor #1	$1,500	1	$1,500	$1,500
	Exhibitor #2	$1,250	1	$1,250	$1,250
			Total Revenues = $14,000		$13,100

WORKSHEET 4.1 *SAMPLE BUDGET WORKSHEET FOR LEARNING ACTIVITY*

And speaking of a yearly budget, the professional development specialist shouldn't limit budget thinking simply to how much can be spent on individual learning activities. The staff educator might need to have his or her own budget to manage, especially if data can be used to demonstrate return on investment. While you're thinking about implementation, jot down guesstimates for the amount of time you spend planning, implementing, and evaluating as well as the time learners spend in class along with their materials, refreshments, and so on (we'll talk more about this in Chapter 6, "Evaluating an Educational Program's Performance").

Deciding on a Format

What type of format you use to deliver a learning activity largely depends on the budget and the educational material used. There are several formats to consider, each meeting different learning needs. The ultimate goal is to plan a learning activity that has a variety of formats included to meet multiple learning styles (see Chapter 2 for a refresher on those, if needed). Online modules, lecture, case scenarios, simulation, group discussions, games, and role play are all examples of formats that you can utilize when planning education. Table 4.5 summarizes the advantages and disadvantages of the various formats.

TABLE 4.5   *ADVANTAGES AND DISADVANTAGES OF COMMONLY USED LEARNING ACTIVITY FORMATS*

FORMAT	ADVANTAGES	DISADVANTAGES
ONLINE MODULES	Self/student paced	Learners in a passive role
	Can be completed around work schedule	No interaction with the instructor
	Good for large learning groups	Technology dependent
LECTURE/ SLIDESHOW PRESENTATION	Instructor control	Learners in a passive role
	Present facts and concepts in a relatively short timeframe	One-way communication
		Pace of learning is controlled by instructor
	Meets auditory learning style	
	Good for large groups of learners	
CASE STUDIES/ SCENARIOS	Encourages critical-thinking skills	Learners need some time to prepare
	Easy to create	May be difficult to find an appropriate case study
	Can be incorporated in other teaching modalities (specifically, simulation or lectures)	Not as effective for large groups

TABLE 4.5 *(CONTINUED)*

FORMAT	ADVANTAGES	DISADVANTAGES
SIMULATION	Controlled/safe representation of reality	Time consuming to plan and implement
	Allows learners to practice problem-solving skills	Cost involved to implement (if using moderate or high-fidelity simulators)
	Allows learners to practice hands-on skills	Can be intimidating for some learners
	Improves communication skills and team building	Allows for domination by one or two learners in a group
	Immediate feedback and evaluation can be provided	Requires a facilitator
	More effective in small groups	
DISCUSSIONS	Learner is in control	Time consuming
	Learners validate their knowledge and skills	Requires a facilitator
		Allows for domination by one or two learners in a group
	Allows instructor to evaluate learning	
	Attitudes can change during discussion	Requires ground rules
	More effective with small groups of learners	Not as effective with large groups of learners
GAMING	Interesting and challenging to students	If too competitive, reduces the focus on learning
	Develops team-building skills	Can intimidate students and create feelings of inadequacy
	Can evaluate learning and provide immediate feedback	
ROLE PLAY	Adds reality to lesson	Can be more focused on the acting versus the concepts
	Builds confidence	
	Focus is on problem solving	Intimidating to some learners
	More effective with small groups	

When considering what will be needed for a learning activity, organize needs into buckets and create a checklist of items needed for the learning activity. Examples of buckets include AV Equipment, Registration Needs, Participant Tools, Classroom Needs, Phone

Numbers, Office Supplies, and Extras. Examples of supplies needed for each bucket are included in Table 4.6.

TABLE 4.6   *WHAT IS NEEDED FOR A LEARNING ACTIVITY*

AV Equipment	Registration Needs
Laptop	Sign-in sheets for participants who registered; blank sign-in sheets for walk-in registrants
Projector	
Projector screen	Receipts for walk-in registrants
Power cords/Duct tape	Pens for sign-in sheets
Computers needed for participants	List of registrants with outstanding balances/payment (if fees associated with activity)
Pointer/Clicker	
Lavalieres	
	Printed out name badges and blanks for walk-in registrants
	Name badge holders
	Signage for sign in and evaluation paperwork
	Evaluation tools if using paper or Scantron evaluations
Participant Tools	**Classroom Needs**
Handouts	Flipcharts
Folders	Markers
Jump drives with slide presentations	Sticky notes for parking lot questions
	Simulation aids, such as simulators/manikins, IV arms, IV poles/pumps
	Equipment used in simulations; for example, dressing kits or trach care kit
Phone Numbers	**Office Supplies**
Speakers	Staplers
AV equipment "Help" desk	Paper clips
Caterers (if used)	Pens
	Pencils (for paper evaluations)
	Tissues
Extras	
Snacks	
Drinks	
Table decorations	

We would encourage you to use this table as a checklist at your next learning activity. Feel free to add to it or modify it to meet your needs.

THE ADVANTAGES OF CHECKLISTS

Checklists are actually useful for far more than simply implementing a learning activity. In fact, the importance of checklists cannot be overstated. Checklists for every aspect of the ADDIE model and the resulting education should be created and used every time. If you use checklists for the mundane as well as the complex activities for which you are responsible, then you are free to think. You can be innovative, take risks, and be able to spend time figuring out how to integrate new education into current practice, strategic goals, and even meeting the Triple Aim. When you spend your mental energy trying to remember all the supplies to bring to a learning activity, you get bogged down in all of the minutiae and end up not being productive.

The Implementation Worksheet

Worksheet 4.2 summarizes each of this chapter's tables into an easy-to-use worksheet that you can reference as you work to implement your learning activity or program.

Conclusion

Education is such a priority for nurses. With the changing dynamic of our patient populations, patient acuities, and the introduction of new technology daily, it is difficult for the professional development specialist to keep up. Learners have high expectations of the product that educators produce. Learners expect education to be relevant to their practice and succinct. They want the flexibility of completing their education during working hours. Learners want a logical structure of the learning activity and the learning materials. Learners also want the opportunity to practice skills and the ability to apply the skills learned into their practice. Learners insist on consistency and subject matter experts in providing the education. Taking a systematic approach when developing educational activities by using the *who, what, when, where,* and *why* when designing the learning activity will assist in keeping the educator organized, focused, and timely as the design and development phases transition to implementation.

	Component	Questions to Ask
Why	Rationale	What is the reason for this learning activity? (Should relate directly back to the Analysis phase [for example, practice gaps, staff concerns, regulatory requirements])
	Promotion to Learners	How will you promote the activity to learners to gain their buy-in? (For example, one-sentence summary, full explanation, sharing full details of practice gaps)
Who	Disciplines	Which disciplines will comprise the target audience? (For example, RNs, UAPs, physicians, social workers)
	Internal versus External	Which units or departments will you invite? Will the activity be limited only to your organization?
	Presenters	Who will be your presenter(s)/facilitator(s)?
When	Timing	When will the event occur, and have I included all relevant stakeholders (for example, learners and facilitators) in determining the time?
	Timeline	How will I organize the timeline for all activities preceding and immediately following the activity? How much flexibility is included for unexpected events?
Where	Location	Where will the activity occur (for example, patient care area, classroom), and what will be needed to make that location conducive to the learning activity (for example, AV equipment, simulators)?
What	Budget/Expenses	How much will the learning activity cost? Consider honorarium, travel and lodging for speakers, printing of brochures/flyers and posters/graphics, program materials and supplies (handouts/folders/jump-drives, etc.), AV rental costs, catering expenses, office supplies (name tags, pens, pencils, paper clips, staplers, receipts), cost of paying staff to attend required learning activities (non-clinical time) and any overtime costs to cover patient care on the nursing unit, sponsors or vendors supporting the program. Also consider whether staff or unit budgets will be required to pay for the educational opportunity. If so, what will that fee cover and how much will the fee be?
	Format	What will the format of the activity be? (For example, online modules, group discussions, games, and so on)
	Supplies	What do I need to bring? AV equipment, registration needs, participation tools, classroom needs, phone numbers, office supplies, and extras (Refer to Table 4.6 for specific items within each of these categories.)

WORKSHEET 4.2 *ASKING THE 5 W'S OF A LEARNING ACTIVITY*

Questions for Reflection/Discussion

1. What tools do you have at your disposal to assist you in meeting all of the development details when designing a learning activity?

2. What resources as far as location, equipment, and materials do you have available to design a learning activity?

3. How can you develop learning activities utilizing multiple formats to meet differing learning styles?

> **KEY TAKEAWAYS**
>
> - *Adult learners link knowledge with past experiences and are problem centered. Providing rationale related to the learning activity allows learners to "buy in" or integrate new knowledge into their practice. This rationale is especially relevant when the learning activity relates to patient safety.*
> - *Consider your target audience—one learning activity does not meet all multidisciplinary needs. Consider creating individualized education for each discipline so the information is succinct and applicable to practice.*
> - *You, as the educator, do not need to be the subject matter expert (SME) for every learning activity. Use your resources and your "true" SMEs to develop and deliver the content. You, as the educator, can use your expert skills in the planning of the learning activity.*

Resources

Puetz, B. E. (1992). The needs assessment: The essence of staff development programs. In K. Kelly, *Nursing staff development: Current competence, future focus*. Philadelphia, PA: J. B. Lippincott.

References

American Association of Critical-Care Nurses. (2012). Timeline for implementing educational programs.

American Nurses Credentialing Center. (2014). *The importance of evaluating the impact of continuing nursing education on outcomes: Professional nursing practice and patient care*. Retrieved from http://www.nursecredentialing.org/Accreditation/ResourcesServices/Evaluating-the-Impact-CNE-Outcomes.pdf

Cincinnati Children's Hospital Medical Center. (2014). Timeline for implementing educational programs.

Cronenwett, L., Sherwood, G., Barnsteiner, J., Disch, J., Johnson, J., Mitchell, P., . . . & Warren, J. (2007). Quality and safety education for nurses. *Nursing Outlook*, 55(3), 122–131. Retrieved from http://www.nursingoutlook.org/article/S0029-6554%2807%2900062-0/fulltext

CHAPTER 5

Evaluating an Individual's Growth

Introduction

At this point in the process, you have analyzed the problem, determined it could be solved with one or more educational activities, designed and developed a structured activity that leverages important learning concepts, and delivered it to the learners. So, you're done, right? Unfortunately, no, you have one more very important piece of the process to perform—evaluation. Evaluation is intended to answer questions like:

- What change(s) resulted from the learning activity?

- How much change resulted from the learning activity?

- Did the learning activity solve (or at least begin to alleviate) the problem that initiated the need for this learning activity?

This chapter and Chapter 6, "Evaluating an Educational Program's Performance," describe the two types of evaluation that staff educators should perform—that of an individual and that of the learning activity or educational program. This chapter starts with the individual level because we as nurses have worked with a lot of people, and it's a bit more natural for us to evaluate an individual's competency, growth, and success than that of a large educational program. At the individual level of evaluation, we might ask targeted questions such as the following:

- Did the individual learner benefit from this learning activity? If so, how? If not, why?

- Is the learner able to perform the necessary job-required activities?

- Is the learner growing and developing as a professional?

Evaluation of a learning activity, even at the individual level, will assist you in determining whether or not the activity successfully achieved its purpose. Hopefully, the evaluation confirms that all of your hard work paid off and that learners are growing and becoming more competent. But even if the evaluation confirms the activity was unsuccessful, it is beneficial for you to know why the learning activity was ineffective so that you can modify and improve (or perhaps remove) that activity for future learners.

You'll notice this chapter is titled "Evaluating an Individual's *Growth*" rather than "Evaluating an Individual's *Competency*." We want to bring attention to two complementary aspects of professional development by acknowledging and promoting that as professional development specialists, we are responsible for not only ensuring our staff are *competent* to perform the job duties required of them but also that they *grow* as professionals in their field.

The growth component begins to move into the realm of managers and mentors who assist staff in their professional development journey, but many of the learning activities staff educators provide will help staff members move beyond basic competency to more advanced knowledge, skills, and attitudes (KSAs). This chapter explores a variety of methods for evaluating both competency and professional growth. The focus is on the former, but as you'll see, there is some overlap.

What Is Competency?

Competency can be (and has been) defined in many different ways, and both organizational leaders and researchers have their own spin on what it entails. We would like to use a simple definition for our purpose here: *Competency* is the ability of an individual to perform the job tasks and duties for which he or she is hired. Regardless of your work setting or organizational policy, this generic definition should be easy to understand. Because competency focuses on those tasks and duties listed upon hire, it can be helpful to have a copy of the job description available for reference. This job description can serve as a gold standard against which to compare whether or not the learner is competent (whether that's to help a preceptor evaluate success during orientation or to assist a manager during performance management).

To describe the various approaches to assessing and ensuring competency, this chapter examines the following considerations:

- Using learning domains (cognitive, psychomotor, and affective) to assess and teach

- Understanding competence versus confidence

- Differentiating nursing skills and personal skills

- Recognizing the novice-to-expert continuum (Benner, 1982)

- Setting goals and making learning plans

Let's start with the most straightforward and practical approach to evaluating competency—by discussing learning domains. As you start reading through the next section, if you've been working in professional development for a while, you might quickly begin to think of situations you experienced that were not as clean-cut as those outlined here. We cover several of those special situations in the subsequent sections, so bear with us as we talk about the ideal world first.

Using Domains of Learning to Assess and Teach

Perhaps the simplest and most structured method of evaluating an individual's competence is by thinking of activities necessary for adequate job performance as falling into three domains: cognitive, psychomotor, and affective. (These are the same three domains used in the world of teaching and learning and that were described in Chapter 3.) They can be simply expressed in evaluation questions such as the following:

- **Cognitive.** Has the learner demonstrated that he or she knows a sufficient amount to safely care for patients?

- **Psychomotor.** Has the learner successfully performed skills that demonstrate the ability to safely care for patients?

- **Affective.** Are the learner's words and actions congruent with the values and beliefs of both the organization and the patient population?

Let's take a look at each of these domains in more detail. A summary of teaching/learning strategies and methods of measurement are shown in Table 5.1, found later in this chapter.

Cognitive Knowledge

Cognitive knowledge is that information you keep inside your head and involves remembering, thinking, problem solving, prioritizing, and reasoning. This knowledge can be a collection of facts and perceptions along with how you arrange that information to make decisions. For example, a nurse leverages cognitive knowledge when viewing laboratory results, recognizing abnormal values, and deciding to notify the physician.

Assessment within this domain should answer the question "Has the learner demonstrated that he or she *knows* a sufficient amount to care safely for patients?" Staff educators measure cognitive knowledge acquisition by using verbal or written evaluation methods.

Psychomotor Skills

Building upon cognitive knowledge, *psychomotor skills* involve a hands-on performance of activities (for example, inserting an intravenous catheter or changing a dressing). Teaching and learning can occur with some of the same strategies as cognitive knowledge, but most learners will prefer being able to practice the skills before performing them on an actual patient. Many nurses claim hands-on training as their preferred learning style, and efforts should be taken by the staff educator to include these skills as often as resources allow. In addition to providing a better match between learning styles and teaching styles, this approach allows a more accurate representation of expected performance in the real world than methods evaluating only cognitive knowledge.

Assessment within this domain should answer the question "Has the learner successfully *performed* skills that demonstrate the ability to care safely for patients?"

Affective Thoughts and Behaviors

Affective knowledge involves a person's values, beliefs, and motivation, and because these are fairly intangible attributes, educators and learners alike often find affective competence to be the most challenging of the three learning domains. Evaluation in this domain answers the question: "Are the learner's words and actions congruent with the values and beliefs of the learner, organization, and the patient population served?"

Methods for teaching/learning and evaluating in this domain include case studies, group discussion, and guided reflection. One beneficial property of all three approaches is that you can develop and use a single scenario and accompanying questions for each of the methods. Consider an example:

> *The family members of a terminally ill patient are requesting a change in advanced directives. The patient had previously signed a do-not-attempt-resuscitation order before being hospitalized, and due to his weakening condition, he is no longer able to competently make medical care decisions. The family members insist on an escalation of care that includes invasive ventilation to assist with breathing. You are the nurse caring for the patient.*
>
> - *How would you handle this situation?*
> - *What do you anticipate your conversation with the family members will be like?*
> - *Will you treat them differently than other visitors?*
> - *How should/would the care of the patient be different?*
> - *What support systems have you identified for yourself to help you through this situation?*

You could use the scenario and guiding questions as a case study for individuals to complete or as a facilitation script for group discussion, or you could ask learners to reflect on the case and compose their answers in a journal-like entry.

A Summary of the Learning Domain Strategies and Evaluation Methods

Check out Table 5.1 for some examples of teaching/learning strategies and accompanying evaluation methods related to each of the domains.

TABLE 5.1 *TEACHING/LEARNING STRATEGIES AND COMPLEMENTARY EVALUATION METHODS FOR EACH LEARNING DOMAIN*

LEARNING DOMAIN	TEACHING/ LEARNING STRATEGIES	EVALUATION METHODS
Cognitive Knowledge	Instructor-led classes	Tests and quizzes
	Online modules	Question and answer discussions
	Assigned readings	
	Observation of experienced nurses in the clinical setting	Documentation reviews
		Case studies
Psychomotor Skills	Observation of experienced nurses in the clinical setting	Direct observation of skill
	Simulation scenarios or skills laboratories	Achievement of desired outcome (for example, verifying correct placement of feeding tube even though you did not observe the tube being placed)
	Online modules (especially if they contain pictures and/or videos)	
Affective Thoughts and Behaviors	Case studies	Evaluate during the teaching/learning strategies on the left
	Group discussion	
	Guided reflection	

Now that we have briefly covered the basics on how you might approach evaluating an individual, let's jump into some of these gray areas. You will still use the same methods listed in Table 5.1 of the previous chapter (for example, quizzes, direct observation, and group discussion), but there will be some additional considerations you will judge.

Differentiating Between Competence and Confidence

As you begin to evaluate an individual's competence in your role as a professional development specialist, you first want to make sure you're evaluating the objective form of competence—that is, an assessment of whether an individual can perform the job tasks and duties for which he or she was hired. There are times where an individual might believe he or she can perform these tasks and duties when in actuality, he or she cannot. In this case, we have confidence without competence.

RECOGNIZING CONFIDENCE WITHOUT COMPETENCE

There are a few phrases that might clue you into questioning whether one is displaying confidence without competence:

- *"I'll be fine. It's not a big deal."*
- *"I didn't score well on that quiz because I'm not a good test-taker."*
- *"I do it perfectly when I'm in the patient's room—I just don't like being observed in the skills lab when you're waiting for me to make a mistake."*

Let's say that *competence* is the degree to which someone is able to practice nursing safely under various conditions (measured by objective tools or other healthcare providers' observations), whereas *confidence* is the self-assessed or perceived degree to which someone is able to practice nursing safely under various conditions. More accurate labels would probably be *subjective (self) competence* (instead of confidence) and *objective competence* (instead of competence). This labeling recognizes the value of the individual in assessing competence.

Note that subjective competence and objective confidence are not mutually exclusive—both could be present or absent in an individual, or they could both be present in varying degrees along a continuum. But to keep things simple, take a look at Table 5.2, which highlights the four possible combinations of these two components and what you might expect in a learner. If you're familiar with the Conscious Competence Theory (described well by Gordon Training International [2011] and BusinessBalls [2015]), these concepts might look somewhat similar.

The most preferable scenario is when objective competence and subjective competence are both high—in this case, you can easily document that competency has been achieved. If objective competence is high, but subjective confidence is low, things will likely turn out fine. You see this scenario in orientees as well as in situations where a new skill or piece of equipment has been introduced into the workplace. With time and practice, one's confidence increases. You might also see some learners described in the lower-right corner of Table 5.2 in those situations where new skills have recently been introduced.

If the nurse has had adequate time to learn new knowledge or skills yet both objective competence and subjective competence are low, the nurse might need to consider finding a more suitable environment. Hopefully, nurses in this situation were identified with this problem while in orientation; however, if they are working independently with low objective competence and low subjective competence, you would want to get the manager involved early to discuss appropriate professional development plans for this nurse.

If you encounter a situation where you're questioning whether subjective competence might be present in the absence of objective competence, you first want to assess the learner's responsiveness to feedback. If this is someone who does not readily receive constructive feedback, you might have a performance issue rather than a learning issue and would consider involving the manager. All of us have room to learn and develop, and for those who are too confident to realize that, working in healthcare might be a challenge. However, if you believe the person is open to feedback, have someone the learner trusts (whether that's you or someone else) approach him or her privately to discuss the observed concerns.

TABLE 5.2   COMPARISONS OF VARIOUS COMBINATIONS OF COMPETENCE AND CONFIDENCE

		COMPETENCE (OBJECTIVE)	
		HIGH	**LOW**
CONFIDENCE (SUBJECTIVE)	High	Demonstrates that both the individual and others agree that competence has been achieved. The nurse can safely perform job duties and tasks under a variety of conditions. Action: Allow the nurse to perform duties and tasks autonomously.	The nurse's perception of his or her performance is greater than that of others' perceptions. This is especially problematic in the event that a learner is not receptive to feedback. Action: Provide open and honest feedback to the nurse. Ensure all stakeholders understand expectations for demonstrating competency. Encourage reflection on performance.
	Low	The nurse is practicing safely but doubts his or her own abilities (more common for less-experienced nurses). This could be problematic if the fear or anxiety is so great that errors occur due to emotional distress. Action: Focus on performance so far, reaffirm strengths, offer to be present when the nurse is performing a task for the first time in a patient care area, and encourage peers to provide praise.	Demonstrates that both the individual and others agree that competence has not been achieved. The nurse is either (a) still actively learning or (b) unfortunately working in an environment that may not be a good fit for his or her skill level and interests. Action: Repeat, modify, or add learning activities if active improvement is demonstrated. Consider transfer or termination if environment is not a good fit.

Source: Adapted from Staff Educator's Guide to Clinical Orientation (Jeffery & Jarvis, 2014).

Distinguishing Between Nursing Skills and Personal Skills

As you evaluate individual learners, you will likely, from time to time, encounter instances where a person may be able to pass a learning activity's test, successfully perform the clinical skills in the simulation lab, and contribute meaningfully in discussion with peers. That is, the evaluation shows that the individual essentially meets all the objective criteria defined as necessary for success. But you feel something is missing and hear phrases like the following:

- "I just can't put my finger on it."
- "He just isn't getting *it*." (And "it" is hard to define.)
- "She can't connect the dots."
- "He's really nice, *but...*."

We believe these situations tend to occur due to two major problems: poor interpersonal communication and an inability to think critically. According to all of the previously mentioned evaluation tools, the learner is succeeding, but the observations of peers, patients, or other bystanders raise concerns about performance. These skills of interpersonal communication and critical thinking are necessary for nurses, but they are difficult to teach and objectively evaluate.

The real world of healthcare is a complex and constantly evolving environment that needs clinicians who can be responsive to the changing needs of the patients and the system as a whole. Interpersonal communication and critical thinking are the underlying skills that help connect and apply the cognitive knowledge, psychomotor skills, and affective thoughts and behaviors to patient care. There are a variety of additional ways we could describe these terms, and many books and articles have been published with that goal. We'll save you the hair-splitting and turn to some approaches we have used when trying to help learners grow in their interpersonal communication and critical thinking.

Interpersonal Communication

If a nurse were to make rude or inappropriate comments to a patient's family member, you would likely question that nurse's affective competency. Overcoming such blatant interpersonal communication issues was addressed in the previous sections. However, there are some more subtle interpersonal communication skills that can make other competencies difficult to evaluate. Some opposing traits include:

- **Taciturn.** Some people are naturally less verbal than others. These people might sometimes be described, albeit inappropriately, as shy, timid, antisocial, or introverted. However, simply because a person doesn't *talk* as much as others does not mean he or she is less competent than someone else or even that the person is less confident. Unfortunately, it can make it difficult to evaluate competency if you don't hear from the person. Make sure you encourage these learners to speak up when they are being evaluated. Helping them understand that it's difficult for an evaluator to assess their knowledge will frequently motivate them to be more communicative during these times.

- **Verbose.** On the opposite side of taciturn are those people who use many words when fewer might do. We're choosing not to use words like *extroverted* and *talkative* because they can have different meanings in different situations. What we're trying to illustrate with a verbose learner is someone who naturally uses a lot of words to express oneself, and unfortunately, it appears to others that he or she does not have clarity of thought. It can be challenging to parse out someone who is unable to succinctly respond to a question because the person doesn't know the answer versus someone who is just naturally verbose. Just as you would explain evaluation challenges to a taciturn learner, you would tell the verbose learner of the challenge in evaluation. Tell these learners it is important for evaluation reasons that they provide succinct responses so that you are able to assess their ability to organize their thoughts and provide prompt responses to clinical situations.

In yet other situations a person's verbal (or even nonverbal) communication makes evaluation a challenge. Always communicate openly with the learners by expressing the challenge the *evaluator* is having in performing the evaluation; the goal is to ensure an objective evaluation, not criticize someone's personal communication strategies. If, however, someone's communication strategies prove to be a challenge to more than just competency evaluation, a focus on strengthening that person's emotional intelligence should prove beneficial.

LEARNING MORE ABOUT EMOTIONAL INTELLIGENCE

Emotional Intelligence (EI) is comprised of four pillars: self-awareness, self-management, social awareness, and relationship management (Goleman, 2006). The focus is on how one perceives and interacts with oneself and others. For some additional information, you could check with your Human Resources department, or here are a few nursing-specific articles that may be of help:

- *Emotional Intelligence: A Review of the Literature With a Specific Focus on Empirical and Epistemological Perspectives, by Kristin Akerjordet and Elisabeth Severinsson (2007)*
- *The Heart of the Art: Emotional Intelligence in Nurse Education, by Dawn Freshwater and Theodore Stickley (2004)*
- *Emotional Intelligence in Nursing Work, by Anne C. H. McQueen (2004)*

Critical Thinking

If you are seriously questioning a learner's critical-thinking ability, there are a few nice formal tools available for evaluating critical thinking (for example, the Health Sciences Reasoning Test [Insight

Assessment, 2013] or the Watson-Glaser Critical Thinking Appraisal [Pearson, 2015]). However, what you *do* in response to the result of such an assessment tool might be limited. For example, just because someone scored low on a critical-thinking test doesn't mean you should (or even could) terminate his or her employment. So, we wouldn't necessarily recommend these tools unless you're developing some new interventions and want to see if those interventions can enhance critical thinking over time.

SITUATIONAL JUDGMENT TESTS

Another option for assessing critical thinking would be to create a situational judgment test, which is a tool that asks respondents how they would react in a specific situation. Although this type of assessment doesn't have the validity and reliability of a more formal test, it could help you establish that the concerns expressed about the learner are, in fact, legitimate concerns. If you haven't worked with situational judgment tests before, check out the following example question and then review the possible—situational—actions a nurse might take based on his or her judgment:

> *You are caring for a patient with severe hypertension in an intensive care unit. The prescribing provider orders a dosage of an antihypertensive that you believe is too high and could result in an unsafe drop in blood pressure. You express your concern to the prescribing provider, who responds that recent literature suggests the prescribed dosage is safe. On a scale of 1 to 5, how appropriate are each of the following actions?*
>
> *a. Refusing to administer the medication*
>
> *b. Administering the medication at a lower dosage than prescribed*
>
> *c. Administering the medication as prescribed*
>
> *d. Calling the charge nurse, manager, or pharmacist for assistance*
>
> *e. Looking up the correct dosage in the pharmacy's formulary*
>
> *f. Increasing blood pressure monitoring frequency following medication administration*

In this kind of test, the "right" and "wrong" answers aren't clear; rather, they require prioritization and judgment under uncertainty. Every patient encounter is somewhat unique, and these situational judgment tests you create can help you to mimic that. Because there aren't typically specific right and wrong answers (except for maybe [b] in the example, which is illegal in most states), these tests can give you insight into how the learner perceives the world and provide you with a safe environment to discuss any discrepancies.

Individuals who are able to pass nursing school and the organization's orientation program typically don't experience any major problems associated with critical thinking. Such problems can exist, however. Table 5.3 provides one approach staff educators can use to evaluate and manage this possibility. This approach is known as the OPQRST (objectivity, patterns, qualify and quantify, reframe and share, and trial) process.

TABLE 5.3   *OPQRST PROCESS FOR APPROACHING STRUGGLES WITH CRITICAL THINKING*

COMPONENT	DESCRIPTION	RATIONALE
OBJECTIVITY	Explore objective accounts of concerning behaviors.	Presuming what the learner is *thinking* before observing what he or she is *doing* could lead to inaccurate conclusions
PATTERNS	Look for a pattern or theme that occurs across multiple scenarios.	Assists with discovering the underlying problem while also considering the potential for situation-dependent factors
QUALIFY AND QUANTIFY	Qualify and/or quantify the impact these patterns could have on patient care.	Measuring impact will help you determine the severity of the problem but will also provide an answer to the "So what?" question if the learner asks
REFRAME AND SHARE	Help the learner look at the situation from a different perspective (reframe) by sharing the emerging pattern or theme with the learner.	Raises the learner's awareness of the problem (although, he or she likely is aware of the problem) and helps explore why the learner proceeded the way he or she did
TRIAL	Try alternative methods for approaching situations.	Helps the learner discover that often there is more than one way to approach a situation and can help the learner begin to make appropriate distinctions

Source: Jeffery & Jarvis (2014).

Although evaluation can be quite challenging, there are a few ways staff educators can help grow critical-thinking skills in those staff members who have demonstrated less than desired levels of critical thinking. Here are some examples of interventions that might be helpful for those who could benefit from growing their critical thinking skills:

- Administer case studies that focus on critical-thinking assessment.

- Create simulated scenarios to evaluate and teach desired skills.

- Converse with the learner and explore thought processes through "What if...?" questions. Examples: What if the patient would have had no breath sounds on the right? What if the patient doesn't speak English? What if you were to get an unexpected admission? What if the catheter became clogged?

CRITICAL-THINKING CASE STUDIES

Here are some of our favorite books that include critical-thinking case studies for various patient care environments:

- *Case Studies in Critical Care Nursing: A Guide for Application and Review, by Sheila Drake Melander (2011)*
- *Winningham's Critical Thinking Cases in Nursing: Medical-Surgical, Pediatric, Maternity, and Psychiatric, by Mariann M. Harding, Julie S. Snyder, and Barbara A. Preusser (2013)*
- *Delmar's Case Study Series: Medical-Surgical Nursing, by Gina M. Anker (2011)*
- *Critical Thinking to Achieve Positive Health Outcomes: Nursing Case Studies and Analyses, by Margaret Lunney (2009)*

While concerns about critical thinking deficiencies might frequently surface, a true deficiency is probably quite rare (especially among nursing staff who have completed their academic preparation and organizational orientation). When these problems are identified, however, prompt intervention is necessary to ensure competent care is provided to patients because adequate critical thinking is necessary for the translation of knowledge, skills, and attitudes into practice.

Recognizing the Novice-to-Expert Continuum

Patricia Benner's "From Novice to Expert" article (1982) is considered a foundational piece in describing nursing skill levels, and the model helps inform another aspect of competency—the idea that a nurse cannot be expected to know *everything* at the beginning of his or her career. Benner's model outlines five major stages of skill acquisition: novice, advanced beginner, competent, proficient, and expert.

We bring up this framework and the idea of a continuum of experience level for a few reasons. First, it should serve as a reminder that we are all on a growth journey, hopefully learning something new every day and reminding us that we shouldn't set unrealistic expectations of those early in the continuum. Additionally, for those at the end of the experience level, it might be challenging to evaluate their proposed solutions to a problem within a narrowly defined set of options on a quiz. Providing additional options through which experienced nurses can demonstrate competency could recognize their experience level and make the competency evaluation more enjoyable for them.

Setting Goals and Making Learning Plans

Now that you have a better idea of what competency is and how it's measured, it's time to discuss what happens for someone who demonstrated that he or she is not competent in one or more facets of practice. If an overall assessment (or one or more individual portions of an assessment) indicates a real or potential deficiency in an individual's competency, action must be taken to bring the individual's competency level within the range of acceptable practice standards. And so the process of applying the ADDIE model begins anew—assessing areas for growth; designing, developing, and implementing educational activities; and evaluating competency once again, this time looking for a change.

Ultimately, the manager is the person responsible for competency assessment, and, according to the Centers for Medicare and Medicaid Services (which contains rules followed by almost all healthcare organizations), managers are responsible for the competency of each and every one of their employees (CMS, 2015). Managers may delegate this assessment responsibility to a staff educator or someone who observes an employee more frequently. Educators who have carefully performed a competency evaluation and find that an employee does not meet acceptable competency levels should immediately notify the responsible manager. The reason for this notification is twofold: The manager might have additional information about the employee's current situation that could shed light on why the employee didn't perform successfully, and only the manager (when operating within the policies set by the organization and implemented by Human Resources) can enforce necessary actions, such as mandating the repetition of a learning activity, suspending work, or even terminating the employee.

NOTE

As you work with individuals to ensure competency, don't forget to consider the legal implications of allowing a healthcare provider who does not meet competency levels to practice.

As part of the job of ensuring that individuals meet or exceed competency standards, the manager and staff educator should work together to set expectations and create goals for learners, and the educator should then design, develop, and implement educational activities and perform evaluations that reassess competency. A goal-based learning plan worksheet, like the one shown in Worksheet 5.1, is a useful tool in this process.

FOR STAFF EDUCATORS: KNOWING WHEN TO WORK WITH THE NURSE MANAGER

We keep referring to various activities for which the nurse manager might be responsible, but what are some of these tasks on which you should work with your manager to ensure? For your reference, the following situations might be times you should collaborate with the nurse manager:

- *The manager should be aware of the content of the learning activity, support the dates for implementation of the activity, and incorporate evaluation of the activity in any communication he or she provides to staff (for example, including a question or two at change of shift report).*

- *The manager should understand his or her role in assisting staff members to understand the value of incorporating the new knowledge, skill, or behavior into their daily work. (When education is seen as a one-off, it is rarely adopted into practice, and thus the cycle of re-education continues.)*

- *The manager and educator could make rounds, asking knowledge questions regarding the education and observing the skill and interaction with patient and family. (Skills for interacting with patients and families are certainly an opportunity for role modeling by the manager.)*

- *The manager and educator provide staff with post-implementation, data-based outcome reports following a practice change. In doing so, the manager communicates how the education supports specific strategic goals as well as the Institute for Healthcare Improvement (IHI) Triple Aim.*

For additional guidance of management tasks, you might want to check out Sigma Theta Tau International's books series The Nurse Manager's Guide to....

Due Date	Expectation/Goal	Learning Activities	Evaluation
[Within 3 weeks]	[The learner] will be able to administer medications within 60 minutes of scheduled administration time.	Review "Timely Administration of Medications" policy. Discuss barriers to timely administration with staff educator.	Patient chart reveals that 100% of medications were administered within 60 minutes of scheduled time over a 1-week period.
[Within 2 weeks]	[The learner] will be able to modify the nursing plan of care in response to the changing patient condition.	Seek assistance from resources (for example, peers, charge nurse, educator) after identifying an abnormal patient assessment. Complete assigned critical thinking activity. Explore online skills manual for select tasks (for example, chest tube management or violent patient de-escalation).	Peer observation of increased incidence of [learner] seeking out resources. Charge nurse observation of nursing plan modification. Completion of critical-thinking activity.
[Within 3 weeks]	[The learner] will be able to independently document in the new electronic medical record (EMR).	Observe workflow of a peer who serves as a resource for the new EMR. Practice documentation in the simulated charting environment.	Documentation complete on all patients within 15 minutes of completing shift.

WORKSHEET 5.1 *SAMPLE GOAL-BASED LEARNING PLAN*

Unfortunately, it can be easy to forget the employee's responsibility in assessing competency. The subjective experience of the learner (as described in Table 5.2) is important in determining competency, and, especially when creating a learning plan, employee input is essential. The staff educator and/or manager can develop a draft, but the employee should agree to the plan and might even offer additional learning activities. Frequent and regular follow-up is essential during this time, so the learning plan might also include "soft" due dates for the interested parties to meet and evaluate progress. If evaluation reveals unsuccessful achievement by the final due dates, the manager should determine whether or not the current work environment remains appropriate for the employee.

Although we have presented the learning plans as a tool for setting, documenting, and assessing performance improvement, there is another use—as a professional development tool used for the growth of an individual beyond the minimum expectations. Professional development specialists are commonly asked for guidance in endeavors such as obtaining certification or pursuing an advanced degree. Because these attempts are somewhat long-term goals, it might be helpful to work with the learner in establishing short-term activities that can help guide him or her to the final goal.

RESOURCES FOR SERVING AS A MENTOR

If you're interested in moving into more of a mentorship role to support an individual's growth, here are a few books we recommend:

- *Mentoring Today's Nurses, by Susan M. Baxley, Kristina S. Ibitayo, and Mary Lou Bond (2013)*
- *The Nurse Manager's Guide to Hiring, Firing, & Inspiring, by Vicki Hess (2010)*
- *The Elements of Mentoring, by W. Brad Johnson and Charles R. Ridley (2008)*

Conclusion

After a learning activity has been implemented, it is essential to ensure individual learners have gained the intended knowledge, skills, and/or behaviors of the activity. Evaluation can take on a variety of formats but should align with the delivery medium of the activity and hopefully answer some of the questions that surfaced during the original Analysis phase of the ADDIE model.

If the individual is not able to perform the necessary tasks, prompt collaboration with the manager is warranted to determine the cause of the poor task performance and develop an appropriate action plan. This scenario is neither uncommon nor the end of the road because not all individual learners will benefit from a unique learning activity. In fact, when a staff member is unable to perform a task, this is a great opportunity for the staff development specialist to apply his or her specialized knowledge and creativity to develop a suitable learning activity for an individual.

Questions for Reflection/Discussion

1. In what areas do you see individuals have the most difficulty developing: cognitive knowledge, psychomotor skills, affective thoughts/behaviors, interpersonal skills, or critical thinking? What could you change about your learning activities to help with this?

2. Who is responsible for performing evaluation in your organization (for example, peers, charge nurses, managers, staff educators)? If only one or two groups are involved, what might be the benefits and challenges of including more stakeholders in evaluation?

3. What is the format of your individualized learning plans (if you have a standardized format), and do you have plans available for helping both (a) learners who are not meeting learning objectives and (b) learners who want to grow professionally (for example, to obtain certification or advance through the clinical ladder)?

KEY TAKEAWAYS

- *Evaluating an individual's competency is a multi-faceted process.*
- *Cognitive knowledge, psychomotor skills, and affective thoughts and behaviors should all be considered in evaluating an individual's competency.*
- *If learning objectives are not met, the cause (for example, learning preferences not aligned with learning activity medium, interpersonal communication, etc.) must be determined before developing an action plan.*

Resources

Akerjordet, K., & Severinsson, E. (2007). Emotional intelligence: A review of the literature with a specific focus on empirical and epistemological perspectives. *Journal of Clinical Nursing, 16*(8), 1405–1416.

Anker, G. M. (2011). *Delmar's case study series: Medical-surgical nursing.* Clifton Park, NY: Delmar.

Baxley, S. M., Ibitayo, K. S., & Bond, M. L. (2013). *Mentoring today's nurses.* Indianapolis, IN: Sigma Theta Tau International.

Drake Melander, S. (2011). *Case studies in critical care nursing: A guide for application and review.* Philadelphia, PA: Elsevier.

Freshwater, D., & Stickley, T. (2004). The heart of the art: Emotional intelligence in nurse education. *Nursing Inquiry, 11*(2), 91–98.

Harding, M. M., Snyder, J. S., & Preusser, B. A. (2013). *Winningham's critical thinking cases in nursing: Medical-surgical, pediatric, maternity, and psychiatric.* St. Louis, MO: Mosby.

Harvard Business School Press. (2006). *Giving feedback: Expert solutions to everyday challenges.* Boston, MA: Harvard Business School Publishing.

Hess, V. (2010). *Nurse manager's guide to hiring, firing, & inspiring.* Indianapolis, IN: Sigma Theta Tau International.

Johnson, W. B., & Ridley, C. R. (2008). *Elements of mentoring.* New York, NY: Palgrave Macmillan.

Lunney, M. (2009). *Critical thinking to achieve positive health outcomes: Nursing case studies and analyses.* Ames: IA: Wiley-Blackwell.

McQueen, A. C. H. (2004). Emotional intelligence in nursing work. *Journal of Advanced Nursing, 47*(1), 101–108.

Nilson, L. B. (2010). *Teaching at its best.* San Francisco, CA: Wiley.

Patterson, K., Grenny, J., McMillan, R., & Switzler, A. (2002). *Crucial conversations: Tools for talking when stakes are high.* New York, NY: McGraw-Hill.

References

Benner, P. (1982). From novice to expert. *The American Journal of Nursing, 82*(3), 402–407.

BusinessBalls. (2015). Conscious competence learning model. Retrieved from http://www.businessballs.com/consciouscompetencelearningmodel.htm

Department of Health and Human Services, Centers for Medicare & Medicaid Services. (2015, January). §482.23(a) Standard: Organization. In *State operations manual*. Retrieved from http://www.cms.gov/Regulations-and-Guidance/Guidance/Manuals/downloads/som107ap_a_hospitals.pdf

Goleman, D. (2006). *Emotional intelligence: The 10th anniversary edition*. New York, NY: Bantam.

Gordon Training International. (2011). Learning a new skill is easier said than done. Retrieved from http://www.gordontraining.com/free-workplace-articles/learning-a-new-skill-is-easier-said-than-done/

Insight Assessment. (2013). Health sciences reasoning test. Retrieved from http://www.insightassessment.com

Jeffery, A. D., & Jarvis, R. L. (2014). *Staff educator's guide to clinical orientation: Onboarding solutions for nurses*. Indianapolis, IN: Sigma Theta Tau International.

Pearson. (2015). The gold standard critical thinking test. San Antonio, TX: Author. Retrieved from http://www.thinkwatson.com/assessments/watson-glaser

Evaluating an Educational Program's Performance

Introduction

Whether you're providing a routine educational program that's offered on a regular basis or a one-time learning activity that was created in response to a specific problem, evaluating the benefit of the program is absolutely essential. Just as the Analysis stage provides you with insight into the need for a learning activity, the Evaluation stage tells you whether additional activities might be warranted. Evaluation of a program's performance is a higher-level overview than evaluating an individual's performance, which Chapter 5 covered. At the program level, staff educators answer questions like the following:

- Was this learning activity beneficial to patients, clinicians, and/or the organization?

- Should we offer this activity again? If so, how might we offer it differently next time?

- Is the benefit of offering this activity worth its costs?

- Was practice change assessed after the learning activity?

- (And just between us staff educators: If someone wanted to get rid of my activity, what could I do to *prove* to the person that doing so would be a bad idea?)

Staff educators might not address all of these questions (at least, not in great depth) for every activity provided, but they should be familiar with the variety of evaluation questions that can be asked and the appropriate situations in which to ask them. In addition to these considerations, educators should consider the tools, time, resources, and data available to them. These topics are discussed in this chapter.

The Importance of Program Evaluation

To see how important evaluation can be, consider the following scenarios.

> **Scenario 1:** Paula was the director of nursing education at a large urban hospital that had a high rate of hospital-acquired pressure ulcers. New prevention and management supplies had been ordered in recent years, but there had been no significant decreases in the pressure ulcer rates. One of the wound care nurses mentioned to Paula that he has observed many direct care providers not using the prevention and management supplies appropriately. Paula initiated a large-scale learning activity that included online modules and a 30-minute hands-on demonstration of appropriate supply use.
>
> Many of the direct care providers and unit-level staff educators were quite upset at the time-consuming burden of mandatory education for something as simple as (in their words) "readjusting a patient's pillow." As the director of nursing education, Paula felt this was the right thing to do but wanted to apply some data to evaluating whether this activity worked. So, she analyzed Supply Chain Management inventory data and discovered the use of supplies had decreased by almost 50% (a big win for the financial

stakeholder). She also analyzed quality improvement reports of pressure ulcer rates for 3 months following the intervention, and already a significant decrease in rates had been noted!

This first example shows how evaluating a variety of outcomes for a learning activity can provide a holistic view of the activity's impact.

Scenario 2: Ken was the new inpatient, nursing educator of a small, critical-access hospital. As a new educator, he began to question several of the annually required activities expected of all nursing staff. During the week of their annual skills fair, for example, all nurses were required to attend an 8-hour inservice for performing high-risk interventions, such as chest tube management, ventilator supervision, and peritoneal dialysis, among others. However, due to recent restructuring of the organization, these skills were only performed on two of the eight units in the hospital.

Ken evaluated last year's skills fair by asking nurses how frequently they performed each of the activities in the past 12 months. Because the only nurses who performed these skills were found in the two previously mentioned units, Ken removed this requirement for nurses from the other six units, and the required educational pay time was decreased. In the event the expertise for these skills were needed in the other units, Ken also posted just-in-time information in the procedure manual along with the phone numbers of the units where trained staff regularly work.

The preceding example shows how the structure of regularly scheduled learning activities might need to change as organizations' (and patients') needs change. Regular evaluation of routinely schedule activities is necessary to prevent wasting time and resources on unnecessary programs.

As we begin this discussion of program-level evaluation, let's start with a word of caution regarding a small pitfall we frequently observe. If you read our first book on orientation, you might remember us mentioning that in the ideal world, the type and form of evaluation used for a program should relate directly to the assessment data that prompted the program's creation. However, what is more commonly performed is evaluation at only the satisfaction ("happiness") level of the learners. As we explore throughout this chapter, it is important to measure satisfaction, but the best evaluations at the end of the ADDIE process look a lot like the assessment performed at the beginning of the ADDIE process. Let's start with a clinical example to help illustrate the importance of this concept:

> Consider the case of a patient with pneumonia who is having trouble breathing. The patient is already on continuous pulse oximetry with hypoxemia noted. You intervene by repositioning the patient and applying supplemental oxygen. Which of the following sets of questions would be most valuable for evaluating the effectiveness of your interventions?

QUESTION SET A	QUESTION SET B
On a scale of 0 to 10, how satisfied are you with my ability to reposition you and apply oxygen?	On a scale of 0 to 10, how would you rate your difficulty in breathing?
Do you think your breathing has changed as a result of my repositioning skills?	Is it easier to breathe now?
Would you recommend supplemental oxygen to other patients?	Do you need us to work on additional treatments to help you breathe more comfortably?

Answer: Question Set B.

Hopefully, you can see the relationship among initial assessment data, accompanying interventions, and evaluation methods. In the clinical scenario, nurses can take a problem like dyspnea, initiating treatments and following up with whether or not the dyspnea is still present. Similarly, if there is a performance issue in the organization, and a new educational program were added to address this performance issue, the best evaluation would involve assessing the continued presence of the performance issue—not whether the learners enjoyed the training or scored better on a test. A word of caution, however: Please don't take this statement to the extreme by never measuring learner satisfaction. There is much that can be learned from measuring learner satisfaction, but you don't want to stop at that level.

Now that we have recognized this important consideration, let's talk about all the ways we can evaluate a program.

Levels and Types of Evaluation

Because evaluating a program's performance is no simple feat due to its potential complexity and resource-consuming nature, staff educators would be wise to consider using a framework or model as a guide. Adhering to a model not only helps to keep things simple but also prevents you from getting off track as new data emerges. There are a variety of evaluation models present throughout multiple industries, and it can be a bit overwhelming to pick one. Fortunately, there is an almost "classic" evaluation model that can serve as a core framework on which more complex or specific models can be created. We'll start with that one as a jumping-off point.

Kirkpatrick's Four Levels of Evaluation

Donald Kirkpatrick (1996) developed a model that is both simple and practical, which is likely the reason for its widespread use. There are four levels of evaluation within the model:

- **Reaction.** Known by some as the "happiness factor" or "smiley sheets," *reaction* is the first level of evaluation and pertains to how learners perceive (or *react*) to the learning activity. This level doesn't include any evaluation of knowledge, skill/behavior, or attitude change, and it doesn't include any impact on patient/organizational outcomes. This level is simply a measure of how much the learner liked or disliked all the aspects of the learning activity. These aspects might include content, delivery method, speaker, physical environment, and so on. The goal behind this level of evaluation is to determine the satisfaction of the learner because, typically, a satisfied learner is a better learner (Kirkpatrick, 1996).

- **Learning.** In contrast to the more subjective nature of the first level, the second level (*learning)* seeks to measure the modification of knowledge, skills/behaviors, and/or attitudes associated with the learning activity. Evaluation becomes slightly more complex at this level because you must develop a standard (for example, a test) by which to measure learning (Kirkpatrick, 1996). Many evaluations at this level include quizzes, case studies, or simulations to measure learning.

- **Behavior.** The third level, *behavior*, requires you to evaluate the effect of a learning activity on an individual's behavior in the actual job setting. Evaluations become increasingly complex at this level because the real world is full of challenges and confounding variables that could influence behaviors. However, behavioral change is one of the primary intentions of an educational program, and, without it, you aren't likely to see an effect on patient or organizational outcomes.

- **Results.** When evaluating at the fourth and final level, *results*, you are evaluating the end-products of an educational program (for example, improvements in quality of care, reduction in costs, or decreased harm). Many people, especially administrators, consider this the most important level of evaluation, but Kirkpatrick (1996) points out that it shouldn't be the *only* level of evaluation. Although evaluating results identifies whether the program achieved its final intended purpose, there are many other factors to consider in determining whether a program should be continued as is. For example, what if the learners hate the program so much that they're considering leaving the organization? Or what if you find that learning isn't occurring, and the change in results was actually due to a process change rather than a learning activity? Measuring multiple aspects of a training program is always wise (as long as you have the resources to do so).

The differences between each level of evaluation are compared in Table 6.1. You can see examples of how to apply each of these levels to actual programs in Table 6.2.

Notice that most of these examples from Table 6.2 surround evaluation at a very high level. This particular model and the ones that follow are intended to take the 30,000-foot view of the program. Although individual competency is evaluated as a component of this view (specifically, for the second and third levels of learning and behavior), we are aggregating results from multiple learners here. At this level, we aren't as concerned with some learners doing better or worse than others on pre-test/post-test differences, but we would be concerned if the majority or all of the learners perform poorly. Individual variation is inescapable and should be addressed with individuals as needed (check out Chapter 5 for more information on this topic). The focus of evaluation here is on the learning activity (or program) as its own entity.

TABLE 6.1   DIFFERENCES BETWEEN KIRKPATRICK'S FOUR LEVELS OF EVALUATION

	REACTION	LEARNING	BEHAVIOR	RESULTS
WHO	Learners	Learners	Learners	Patient and/or organization
WHAT	Satisfaction	Knowledge, skills, and/or attitudes	Actions (behaviors)	End-outcomes
WHEN	Immediately following the activity	Ideally, soon after the activity Can also consider pre-activity (as a comparison) or repeated evaluations (to assess retention)	During actual job performance	Can take several months (or even years) to see an effect
WHERE	In the same location as the activity	Dependent on activity	In a real-world setting	Dependent on activity
WHY	Happy learners make better learners	Determines if knowledge, skills, or attitudes were modified	Behavioral change is necessary for improved outcomes	Determines if primary outcome was influenced
HOW	Surveys Likert scales Open-ended responses In-person or group interviews	Pre-test/post-test exams Case studies Self-report	Direct observation Self-report Peer assessment Chart audits	Costs Patient care and quality indicators

TABLE 6.2 *EXAMPLES OF USING KIRKPATRICK'S FOUR LEVELS OF EVALUATION*

SCENARIO

Imagine you are tasked with assessing the effectiveness of an annual, organizational training program that involves infection prevention. This program includes online modules for all types of healthcare-acquired infections and a hands-on demonstration of urinary catheter and central venous catheter maintenance. The following questions are possible measurements that could be used to assess the various levels of evaluation.

Level	Sample Measurements
Reaction	According to a Likert scale (for example, on a scale of 1–5 [from Strongly Disagree to Strongly Agree]) survey, were the learners satisfied with educational content, time allowed to complete the activities, ease of using the online module, and ease of finding a reviewer to assess the hands-on demonstration?
	Based on open-ended/anecdotal feedback from learners, what could be changed about the program to make it better?
Learning	What was the measurable difference between pre-module and post-module quizzes used to assess cognitive knowledge in preventing healthcare-acquired infections?
	In the hands-on *demonstration* (that is, in a simulated setting), can learners who have recently completed the activity perform the necessary skills?
Behavior	In the *actual unit*, can learners who have recently completed the activity perform the necessary skills?
	What progress do managers, educators, and/or experienced peers observe with respect to clinical skills?
Results	Did infection rates change following completion of the learning activity?
	What was the cost of implementing the learning activity?

Other Evaluation Models

Additional models or methods to consider when developing your approach to an evaluation include RSA, CIPP, ROI, and CBR. We break down each of these abbreviations in the following sections.

RSA Model

The RSA Model was developed by Roberta S. Abruzzese (1992) [hence the name] and includes components that are very similar to Kirkpatrick's model:

- Process (learner satisfaction)

- Content (the change in knowledge/skill/attitude acquisition)

- Outcome (performance/behavior changes in the real world)

- Impact (organizational results)

- Total Program (the big picture view incorporating all four previous components)

CIPP Model

The CIPP Model was developed by Daniel L. Stufflebeam (1971; 2007), and while it looks similar to the aforementioned models, it has been particularly useful for program evaluation by external entities (for example, consultants or those not involved in the day-to-day activities). The components include:

- **Context**—Evaluation of the system/environmental factors that influence the educational program

- **Input**—Comparison of the various strategies and resources available to implement the program

- **Process**—Assessment of actual program activities in the real world

- **Product**—Determination of whether goals were achieved and whether the program should be sustained in current form

ROI and CBR Analyses

If you want to talk dollars and cents to beef up your evaluation report, calculating a return on investment (ROI) or cost–benefit ratio (CBR) can be helpful. Although direct care providers might not be as interested, using ROI/CBR data can be particularly beneficial when communicating with senior level management. Both calculations provide similar information, but the formulas are slightly different:

ROI (%) = (Benefits − Costs) / (Costs × 100)
CBR = (Program Benefits) / (Program Costs)

The desired results from these calculations would be to obtain a number greater than or equal to 100% for an ROI or 1 for a CBR. Those values indicate that the benefits (return) of the activity are greater than the costs (investments).

Plan to perform a full ROI analysis once per quarter. This means you need pre-education data related to the learning activity in order to compare it to post-education data after the activity has been implemented. For example, consider a facility that has recently learned that the use of a non-chargeable item as a means of decreasing pressure ulcers has skyrocketed. Using the example from earlier (noted as Scenario 1) in the chapter that examined supply chain management and pressure ulcer rates, how might you perform an ROI?

1. Request a report of usage for a specified period of time (perhaps a month) from supply management personnel that is sorted by unit/department.

2. Request a report of the number of pressure ulcers for the same time period that is also sorted by unit/department.

3. Share these reports with both leadership and staff members.

4. Review the literature to determine best practices for use of supplies in preventing pressure ulcers. Ask the nurse stakeholders (perhaps shared governance representatives) to determine how the product is currently used, and identify criteria (again, with the stakeholders) for when/how the product *should* be used on patients, based upon the evidence.

5. Provide learning activities related to the proper use of the product/supply. Also consider incorporating aspects of patient education, as education should never be a one-off due to the volume of information that the nurse learner must absorb each shift. (We have used "3 times" [see-one, do-one, teach-one] or "3 different ways" [for example, online, skills lab, and supervised] as a baseline for educating on various topics.)

6. Request a usage report (sorted by unit) in a specified period of time and compare results to pre-education reports. (Due to the various schedules of nurse learners, already scheduled education, and so on, we suggest using a 3-month window.)

7. Celebrate those units who followed the new standard criteria for use of the product resulting in cost savings and no increase in pressure ulcers.

8. Work with units that have not decreased product use and/or had an increase in pressure ulcers to identify why the education was not applied in the practice setting.

This example demonstrates how the educator can influence practice, decrease cost, and affect patient outcomes while supporting the facility and the Institute for Healthcare Improvement (IHI) Triple Aim.

You can perform an ROI for activities as complex as the pressure ulcer example or as simple as comparing the time spent in preparing a certification review course and then determining the number of staff members who achieve certification. Does your facility use interactive televisions in patient waiting/hospital rooms? As the staff educator, request that data that are collected be related to the top 10 assigned learning activities to ensure the learners are knowledgeable in the assigned/prescribed content to support the patients and their families.

How to Choose the Right Model

Feel free to mix and match from whichever evaluation frameworks make the most sense to you (see Table 6.3 for a comparison of the advantages and disadvantages). There is no one-size-fits-all approach because each program is likely to have some unique attributes that warrant creative evaluation methods. Additionally, not every level of the aforementioned models is necessary for every learning activity. We want to remind you at this point that the evaluation should be guided by the analysis data that originally identified the need for the educational program. Just as the pain example at the beginning of the chapter identified a problem-specific evaluation method, so too should your choice of evaluation method be guided by the problem at hand.

One of the most important factors to consider is the feasibility or practicality of evaluation methods, given a limited amount of time and other resources. There is probably a fancy framework or formula available to determine this, but we rely on the common sense approach. For example, if it's going to take months of data collection to determine whether your organization saved a few hundred dollars in its annual budget, the time and the expense of a formal evaluation are probably not worthwhile. However, you always want to see if there are data sources available that are already being measured that you can tap into for evaluation. For example, if the organization is already measuring incident rates (for example, pressure ulcers), you can easily use its information in the Results/Outputs/Product section of your evaluation without any additional work (except for finding where the most current data are located).

TABLE 6.3   *COMPARISON OF LEVELS OF EVALUATION MODELS*

LEVEL	PROS	CONS
REACTION/ PROCESS/ CONTEXT	Easy to measure Easy to make quick changes Assists in determining learner satisfaction and motivation	Does not provide an objective assessment of knowledge transfer
LEARNING/ CONTENT/ INPUT	Relatively simple to create the instrument Quick and easy to gather data Provides an objective assessment of knowledge transfer	Does not ensure knowledge is transferred to on-the-job behaviors
BEHAVIOR/ OUTCOME/ PROCESS	Higher level of evaluation that assesses application/ use of training concepts Potentially serves as an opportunity for the observer to correct behaviors in real time	Resource-consuming (time spent observing behavior) Does not ensure the program will have an effect on the desired outcome (for example, patient care or cost-savings)
RESULTS/ IMPACT/ PRODUCT	Likely to be of greatest interest to senior-level leaders who manage the budget and other resources	Complex Resource-consuming (both time and money)

Keeping in mind that the goal of selecting a model is to have a systematic approach to evaluation to determine if you should sustain, discard, or modify your programs, let's see how you can apply these models to your healthcare setting.

Evaluation of Activities and Programs

For discussion purposes, we want to identify two different environments or contexts in which you might evaluate your work (we're trying to stay away from the word "levels" because those are used in the models): an entire educational program and smaller learning activities. Although we have been using phrases interchangeably so far, here we talk about their differences when it comes to evaluation.

Think of *learning activities* as those well-defined individual educational opportunities with which learners engage. These might include a class, inservice, workshop, module, or case study. In contrast, *educational programs* are those larger, more holistic (and perhaps more dynamic) educational undertakings comprised of many smaller learning activities. Figure 6.1 illustrates how we're defining these two terms and provides a real-world example of an educational program and its associated learning activities.

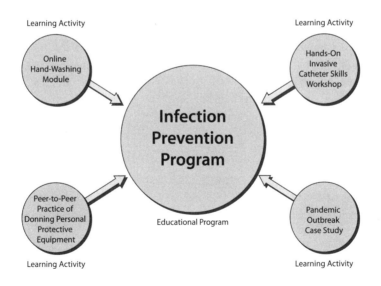

FIGURE 6.1

A Sample of Learning Activities That Make Up the Larger Educational Program

Evaluating an Entire Educational Program

Using Kirkpatrick's model (1996), let's consider doing a global evaluation of an organization-wide educational program. The overall focus of the program could be about infection prevention, safety behaviors, new employee orientation, high-risk equipment skills, medication administration, patient handling, communication, or documentation/charting. Regardless of the topic, type of organization, or who is responsible for overseeing the educational program, the most important consideration in evaluating a program is answering the question: "Does the program meet the needs of the organization while supporting its mission, vision, and values?"

Unfortunately, the answer to this question will be as unique as your organization and the patients it serves.

When thinking about this question, consider some of the evaluation tools at your disposal and how you might evaluate all the aspects of your program systematically, objectively, and feasibly. Make notes of several possible evaluation strategies at all levels in your chosen evaluation model, and keep a record of this. Not only will this help you provide reports for stakeholders, but it will also help you prepare an abstract or publication for sharing your best practice with other staff development specialists in the field.

Evaluating a Learning Activity

Many of the concepts mentioned in evaluating an entire educational program also are applicable to a learning activity. This applicability is especially true if the learning activity is a stand-alone, mini program. For example, let's say your organization performs an annual restraint inservice for its nursing staff. It consists only of an online module that essentially reviews the policy and emphasizes any updates since last year's inservice. If this inservice is not part of any larger program (for example, a Patient Safety and Protection Initiative), you could evaluate this activity as a program as described in the previous section.

However, let's say you do have a larger Patient Safety and Protection Initiative, of which physical restraint is a component. In this case, your evaluation of the restraint learning activity is aimed at *both* its contribution toward the Patient Safety and Protection Initiative as well as the organization as a whole. This change and additional complexity in influence is illustrated in Figure 6.2.

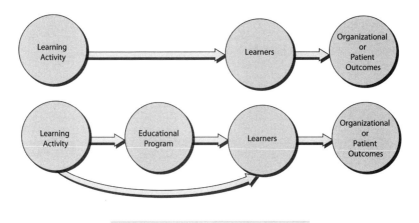

FIGURE 6.2

Learning Activities' Influence on Outcomes

This difference can be important to consider for a few reasons. Have you ever been in a lengthy inservice with multiple presenters where some of the topics were repeated? For example, the how-to's of documenting advanced directives might be covered in both an Electronic Documentation class and an End-of-Life Care class for new employees. If someone were to perform an evaluation of the learning activities of the larger educational program, they might discover the repeated content and consider removing it because the duplicate content could be wasteful. However, what if the repeating of this content was actually the key element in ensuring that learners in the clinical setting really documented advanced directives? Only by evaluating the impact of the activity's removal on organizational/patient outcomes could you definitely say the repeated learning activity isn't necessary.

The "define and discover" approach can be used within the context of a learning activity or an educational program. Worksheet 6.1 shows an example of how to evaluate a learning activity by asking you to define the intentions of the learning activity within an educational program and then to discover how (or even if) the activity achieves its intended purposes.

Define – "What or who is/are…"	Discover – "How does the learning activity…"
…the purpose of the educational program in which the learning activity is found?	…contribute toward the educational program achieving its purpose?
…the gap(s)/need(s) in the educational program?	…address those needs?
…the key stakeholders for the educational program, and what do they want out of the program?	…meet stakeholders' goals and desires?
…other important factors to consider from the needs assessment (performed in Chapter 2)?	…meet the needs identified in the Analysis stage?
Final Question	Final Question
Does the learning activity currently include any other components that are not listed elsewhere?	If the learning activity includes unlisted components, are these components still needed, or should you consider removing them?

WORKSHEET 6.1 *EVALUATING A LEARNING ACTIVITY*

Generic Evaluation Worksheet

Regardless of which setting/context of evaluation you use, when it comes to the level of evaluation and the specific methods, the process becomes more generalized. We have blended several models described in this chapter into an adaptable worksheet (see Worksheet 6.2) to help you specify how you want to evaluate either an entire educational program or a specific learning activity. If you have multiple activities or programs to evaluate, we recommend making a separate worksheet for each.

Component	Questions to Ask
Satisfaction/ Reaction/Process	How will you measure learner satisfaction? (Surveys, Likert scales, open-ended responses, in-person or group interviews, immediately following program versus some time after program, and so on)
Learning/Content	How will you measure the degree to which knowledge, skills, or attitudes were acquired or changed? (pre-test/post-test exams, case studies, self-report, etc.)
Behavior/Outcome	How will you measure performance while in the clinical setting? (Direct observation, self-report, peer assessment, chart audits, and so on)
Results/Impact	How will you measure the unit/organizational impact? (Cost [ROI/CBR], patient care [quality indicators or dashboards], and so on)
Already Measuring	Are there any measures currently being assessed in the organization that could relate to your program? (Quality indicators, length of orientation, and so on)
Who/When	Who is going to collect the data you would like measured, and when are they going to do it?
Other	What other components should be considered in evaluating this program?

WORKSHEET 6.2 *GENERIC EVALUATION WORKSHEET WITH GUIDING QUESTIONS*

Source: Jeffery & Jarvis (2014).

Connecting Evaluation and Analysis

We have mentioned this already, but just to make sure you don't leave this chapter without this in mind… your evaluation methods should correspond to the problems or concerns that surfaced during your analysis that sparked the development of the learning activity or educational program. If rises in medication errors prompted a new learning activity on medication safety, the evaluation would be incomplete without measuring medication error rates. Or if budget cuts resulted in the elimination of an annual skills fair, a proper evaluation would include a measure of the costs associated with this event (in terms of both salary for learners' attendance *and* any adverse events resulting from staff not having this training).

Conclusion

Whether these worksheets seem overly simple or the models seem too abstract, you would be amazed at the number of times we have found benefit in following a systematic approach to evaluating our work. We know that you put sweat, blood, and tears into your learning activities, and we would hate for you to miss out on the opportunity to demonstrate to others the impact your hard work has on learners, organizations, and patients. Using these systematic approaches, regardless of how you do it, will help you ensure you have a beneficial program (while also demonstrating to others that your position is necessary!).

In addition, the record keeping associated with evaluation can help changing leadership personnel or your successors know the story of how a particular program came to be what it is. Rather than everyone having to learn the hard way in trying what they think are new ideas, keep a record of your evaluation to show what worked and what didn't. Some things that didn't work in the past might work now, and it could save the organization a large amount of time and resources to not reinvent the proverbial wheel.

Questions for Reflection/Discussion

1. What processes do you currently have in place for evaluating your educational programs and/or learning activities?

2. Could you use additional models or levels of evaluation to more fully demonstrate the benefit of your learning activities or educational programs?

3. How do you see the use of multiple evaluation methods assisting you in building a case for additional educational resources?

4. How do you currently differentiate between the impact of learning activities and educational programs? How might you differentiate between them moving forward?

5. What resources and barriers are present for activity/program evaluation in your organization?

KEY TAKEAWAYS

- *Evaluating educational programs and associated learning activities is vitally important to an organization's mission, vision, and values.*
- *Review strengths and weaknesses from multiple evaluation frameworks and create something that works for you and your organization.*
- *Perform evaluations regularly and systematically.*
- *Evaluate programs and learning activities at multiple levels to provide a holistic evaluation.*

References

Abruzzese, R. S. (1992). *Nursing staff development: Strategies for success.* St. Louis, MO: Mosby.

Jeffery, A. D., & Jarvis, R. L. (2014). *Staff educator's guide to clinical orientation: Onboarding solutions for nurses.* Indianapolis, IN: Sigma Theta Tau International.

Kirkpatrick, D. (1996). Great ideas revisited: Revisiting Kirkpatrick's four-level model. *Training and Development, 50*(1), 54–59.

Stufflebeam, D. L. (1971, February 24). The relevance of the CIPP evaluation model for educational accountability. Annual Meeting of the American Association of School Administrators. Atlantic City, NJ.

Stufflebeam, D. L. (2007). *CIPP evaluation model checklist* (2nd ed.). Retrieved from http://oceanleadership.org/wp-content/uploads/2011/07/cippchecklist-Attch-2.pdf

CHAPTER 7

Ethical and Legal Considerations

Introduction

The first six chapters focus on introducing the ADDIE model and explaining the various phases of providing nurse learners with education, but with each of these phases comes additional considerations about which the professional development specialist must be aware. These include ethical considerations, accredited continuing education (CE) procedures, certification, professional organization involvement, leadership and confidentiality, and record keeping. Because these topics surface frequently in the practice of a professional development specialist, we designed this chapter to help you be successful in facing the challenges that arise.

Ethics

From the early days of the profession, nurses have always focused on caring for the sick. The American Nurses Association (ANA, 2015b) describes the profession as encompassing "the prevention of illness, the alleviation of suffering, and the protection, promotion, and restoration of health in the care of individuals, families, groups and communities." With this responsibility comes a host of ethical and legal considerations. The staff educator is bound to the same standards as the bedside nurse, which includes the ANA Code of Ethics, accrediting bodies such as The Joint Commission (TJC) and the Centers for Medicare and Medicaid Services (CMS), along with ANA's *Nursing Professional Development: Scope and Standards of Practice* (2010). For the purposes of the chapter, we focus on the ANA Code of Ethics and its implication for the staff educator. The ANA Code of Ethics is the standard guide used to direct the ethical practices of nursing and outlines consistent nursing responsibilities. In case you haven't reviewed them in a while, Table 7.1 identifies the ANA's provisions.

At first glance, many nurses feel the ANA Code of Ethics is only directed to bedside nurses. But the reality is the ANA Code of Ethics is the responsibility for all nurses to uphold, regardless of their position. The staff educator, for example, plays a supportive role in the work of the bedside nurse and is indirectly involved in patient care as a result. Much of the work of the staff educator is to model appropriate behaviors and actions and to provide the resources for bedside nurses so that they can provide the best care possible for their patients.

One aspect of the staff educator role is to serve as part of the leadership team for a nursing unit, and all leaders must model appropriate behaviors consistently with staff members. The following list provides several general examples of how leaders can exemplify ethical behavior:

- Practice respect and kind interactions with patients, families, and colleagues.

- Advocate for appropriate care for patients through interactions with colleagues.

- Develop learning activities based on a needs assessment of the staff.

- Provide a safe environment for patients, families, and colleagues.

- Be respectful of the privacy of patients and families.

- Be respectful of staff privacy.

- Maintain professional boundaries with patients and families.

TABLE 7.1 *ANA CODE OF ETHICS*

PROVISIONS

Provision 1:	The nurse, in all professional relationships, practices with compassion and respect for the inherent dignity, worth, and uniqueness of every individual, unrestricted by considerations of social or economic status, personal attributes, or the nature of health problems.
Provision 2:	The nurse's primary commitment is to the patient, whether an individual, family, group, or community.
Provision 3:	The nurse promotes, advocates for, and strives to protect the health, safety, and rights of the patient.
Provision 4:	The nurse is responsible and accountable for individual nursing practice and determines the appropriate delegation of tasks consistent with the nurse's obligation to provide optimum patient care.
Provision 5:	The nurse owes the same duties to self as to others, including the responsibility to preserve integrity and safety, to maintain competence, and to continue personal and professional growth.
Provision 6:	The nurse participates in establishing, maintaining, and improving healthcare environments and conditions of employment conducive to the provision of quality care and consistent with the values of the profession through individual and collective action.
Provision 7:	The nurse participates in the advancement of the profession through contributions to practice, education, administration, and knowledge development.
Provision 8:	The nurse collaborates with other health professionals and the public in promoting community, national, and international efforts to meet health needs.
Provision 9:	The profession of nursing, as represented by associations and their members, is responsible for articulating nursing values, for maintaining the integrity of the profession and its practice, and for shaping social policy.

Source: ANA (2015b). Code of ethics for nurses with interpretative statements. Retrieved from http://www.nursingworld.org/MainMenuCategories/EthicsStandards/CodeofEthicsforNurses/Code-of-Ethics-For-Nurses.html

Beyond these leader-focused ethical implications is a host of professional development-specific implications of the ANA's ethical provisions. These include:

- Promoting lifelong learning

- Ensuring successful orientation/onboarding

- Setting professional boundaries

- Assessing competence

- Ensuring patient/employee safety

- Facilitating teamwork/delegation

We discuss each of these provisions as they relate to the professional development specialist in the following sections.

Promoting Lifelong Learning

Nurses are lifelong learners. According to the ANA, "Nurses must continue to learn about new concepts, issues, concerns, controversies, and healthcare ethics relevant to the current and evolving scope and standards of nursing practice" (2015b). Evidence-based practice (EBP) changes occur almost on a daily basis. It is the responsibility of the nurse to keep up to date on these practice changes to provide patients with optimal care. Keeping current on all of these changes can be an overwhelming task to bedside nurses. Staff educators support nurses in this task by helping the nurse weed through the changes and bring back to the unit those practice changes that meet the needs of the nurses on the unit and the patients they care for daily.

Educators do so much to support the lifelong learning of bedside nurses so they can best care for patients, and a byproduct of the learning is professional growth and development. Avenues for support include the following:

- General certifications

- Advanced life support certifications (for example, ACLS or PALS)

- Returning to school for degree advancement

- Involvement in professional nursing organizations

- Presenting research and best practice projects in podium or poster presentations

- Attending national and local conferences

- Participating in unit-based and hospital-based shared governance programs and committees

- Becoming successful preceptors and mentors

- Facilitating the successful transition to leadership roles on the unit (for example, charge nurse positions)

- Advancement or lateral moves into other positions within an institution

- Career ladder advancement programs

Ensuring Successful Orientation and Onboarding

The staff educator invests a large amount of time in supporting professional relationships on the nursing unit, especially with new staff members. Unfortunately, many nurses have heard how those in the profession tend to "eat their young" and participate in horizontal violence or hostility in the workplace, commonly known as *bullying*. These behaviors affect so many of our new nurses as they onboard to a nursing unit. This behavior creates a negative work environment and makes it extremely difficult for a new nurse to succeed. Staff educators can create an atmosphere where behaviors of bad-mouthing, gossiping, and harassment are not acceptable. By modeling appropriate behaviors, expecting respect for all team members, and developing team-inclusion and team-building exercises, staff educators can build and maintain healthy professional working relationships.

An additional way to ensure the newly hired absorb and apply these expectations is for the educator to use the ANA Code of Ethics as part of the framework for orientation. The idea is the Code of Ethics statements become expected behaviors for the nurse and the patient, and between nurse to nurse. By doing the following, you can ensure the Code of Ethics statements are incorporated into orientation and onboarding.

- Incorporating the statements from the ANA Code of Ethics into learning activities.

- Incorporating safety aspects whenever and wherever possible. For example, principles of infection control are crucial to safety. Because hand-washing isn't always second nature, practice again and again with the new employee until the learner is asking why you skipped hand-washing as the first step when learning a new procedure.

- Educating orientation session facilitators and speakers on how to incorporate the onboarding competencies and expected learner outcomes into their presentations. Because the newly hired nurse will need to know regulatory requirements and what data his or her care contributes to, such as National Database of Nursing Quality Indicators (NDNQI), it is important for the staff educator to help the speakers make the connection between their content and what is being tracked.

- Educating the managers on onboarding content and learner outcomes for the newly hired nurse. Because the manager is responsible for staff performance, the educator must *communicate* what the onboarding program provides in order for the manager to be able to support and reinforce the content in the clinical setting.

- Educating the preceptors of the newly hired nurse. This is important because the preceptor might not have kept up with the current evidence, or even changes in policy. Whereas the preceptor is responsible for socializing, role modeling, and educating new staff, it is the staff educator who must ensure the preceptors are practicing at the highest level.

TRANSLATING HOW THE ANA CODE OF ETHICS IS PART OF THE ORIENTATION FRAMEWORK

The following list shows how you might communicate how Provision 3 of the ANA Code of Ethics with Interpretive Statements is part of the orientation framework. Provision 3 states, "The nurse promotes, advocates for, and strives to protect the health, safety, and rights of the patient" (ANA, 2015b).

- *Incorporate/review the essentials of the facility's safety program by asking speakers to include subject-specific safety components in presentations, simulations, and online modules.*

- *Discuss how to communicate potential concerns to other health team members, such as medical assistants, patient care assistants, and physical and respiratory therapists. Document concerns where other healthcare members can review and note patient changes in a shift report. Newly hired nurses must learn from the outset the importance of being the coordinator of care, and what that means for keeping patient safety at the forefront of daily practice.*

- *Discuss patient safety as part of patient education. Incorporate return demonstration and application of concepts (teach-back) of planned discharge education into daily practice. It is still the expectation that discharge planning begins upon admission for inpatient visits or during initial interaction during office, urgent care, or emergency department (ED) visits. By starting discharge planning from the beginning of patient contact, nurses can contribute to the prevention of readmissions. Readmissions, you will recall from your "current awareness" of regulatory requirements, is an expectation of the U.S. federal government. Again, the nurse learner is improving patient outcomes and experience as well as decreasing cost to patients and facilities (all of which is part of the Institute for Healthcare Improvement [IHI] Triple Aim).*

- *Educate the preceptors on a standardized way to coach new orientees and the responsibility for assessing the progress of the orientee in an ethical manner.*

- *Weave the importance of the ANA's Professional Role Competence position statement (2014) into orientation.*

Although a great deal of time is spent in the learner's acquisition of skill competency, it is the nurse learner's overall acquisition of knowledge/ skills/attitudes (the three domains of learning) specific to the nursing profession that results in caring behaviors experienced by patients and families. It is how the art of nursing care becomes the practice of nursing.

Previously, we noted the importance of having standard policies, procedures, and practices as the basis for providing safe nursing care to patients. Here, we are stating the importance of using the ANA Code of Ethics as a standard framework for nurse safety. While regulatory agencies and state boards of nursing have specific requirements to guard patient safety, being able to know that all of your nursing colleagues are competent in the basics of what your organization expects, what your leaders expect, what your patients expect, and what your colleagues expect ensures best practice is provided every shift.

Setting Professional Boundaries

Another ethical consideration with which the staff educator can assist learners is through the setting of professional boundaries. You can develop learning activities (we especially recommend discussing case scenarios) to illustrate the importance of maintaining professional boundaries and the ramifications of crossing the line with patients and families. Nurses care for patients at very vulnerable times in their life. Whether patients are hospitalized for short or long periods of time, nurses develop deep relationships with them. Because of the nature of this relationship, personal information is shared and trust is established. Especially as it pertains to establishing contact via social media outlets, it can be very easy for bedside nurses to be placed in uncomfortable situations. Social media makes it easy for patients and families to attempt to continue the relationship, which places nurses in an awkward situation. The staff educator can assist in supporting staff in maintaining professional boundaries by providing opportunities to learn and discuss communication strategies when faced with these situations.

Assessing Competence

The ANA (2015b) explicitly notes that as an advocate for the patient, "the nurse must be alert to and take appropriate action regarding any instances of incompetent, unethical, illegal, or impaired practice by any member of the health care team or the health care system or any action on the part of others that places the rights or best interests of the patient in jeopardy." This accountability directly involves the staff educator and his or her role as a leader on the nursing unit. It is the responsibility of the staff educator to teach, monitor, and evaluate nursing practice as a member of the leadership team. A nurse should not be released from orientation if the nurse is not meeting standard competencies expected during the onboarding process. The decision to release a nurse from orientation is a collaborative decision among the manager, educator, preceptor, and new nurse. Similarly, if a nurse is struggling to achieve or maintain expected competencies, an extension of orientation or a determination if the nurse is a right fit for the practice area should be made by the employee, staff educator, and manager.

The bottom line is that all nurses—including staff educators—need to provide safe and competent care. Educators have an ethical obligation to notify managers if a peer is displaying incompetence, unsafe care, or impairment. If a novice or experienced nurse displays incompetent practice, the manager and educator should determine if more education is needed. If so, a plan of action should be developed by the staff educator and the employee to meet the learning needs of the individual (check out Chapter 5 for an example worksheet on how to do this). If this is not an education issue (for example, the actions displayed are intentional noncompliance with an expected practice), then the burden of responding lies with the manager.

Ensuring the Safety of Patients and Employees

The staff educator promotes and protects the rights, health, and safety of patients and employees by incorporating safety principles into all learning activities. Sharing safe practices as they relate to procedures, new equipment, and changes in treatment modalities brings home the importance of a culture of safety. When developing a learning activity for staff members, staff educators should be creative in considering how to incorporate safety practices into the education. For example, the staff educator should integrate the importance of hand-washing before the start of any patient procedure. Or, in providing an inservice on new intravenous infusion pumps, the educator could discuss the safety features of the device and provide ideas for troubleshooting when the use of the new device doesn't go as planned.

The culture of safety also applies to patient education. Educators should discuss with staff members the importance of routinely including patient safety as part of all patient education. As part of this patient education, educators should encourage and support staff to incorporate return demonstrations, such as teach-back, into daily practice to ensure patients and families are able to correctly and safely complete tasks that they need to continue after discharge.

Facilitating Delegation and Teamwork

As coordinators of care, RNs (whether the frontline providers or the leaders that support those that deliver direct care) are responsible for the quality of care provided to patients. With more and more roles taking additional responsibility for direct patient care, RNs must be accountable for understanding patient needs; knowing who the members of the team are for their shift and what their capabilities are; and determining when, what, and why to delegate to each team member.

Delegation is a key example of a daily task that proves to be a challenge when ensuring the delivery of high-quality care. The staff educator can develop learning opportunities that support the practice of delegation, including appropriate follow-up related to the delegated task. Bedside nurses should have an understanding of what can and cannot be delegated in one's organization and according to that state's nurse practice act. The bedside nurse should feel comfortable with setting parameters for following up on delegated tasks. The staff educator might consider creating team-building exercises to assist in trust building within a multidisciplinary team.

Hopefully, you are beginning to appreciate that the ethical standards by which nurses practice are not limited to a piece of paper or simply the role of direct care providers. The ethical standards permeate all levels of a healthcare organization and have implications for several practice areas of the professional development specialist.

Accredited Continuing Education

Some individuals find it confusing to distinguish between continuing education (CE) and inservices, using the terms interchangeably. Although it might be fine to refer to them interchangeably when talking informally, staff educators need to understand the distinction. *Accredited* CE is designed to augment or enhance the learner's knowledge or skills, whereas *inservices* are designed to review, maintain, or increase expected knowledge and skills related to the learner's job position or the expectation of the institution. Inservices are not eligible for accredited CE hours. For example, orientation, yearly competency reviews, and new equipment inservices are not eligible for accredited CE. However, topics like new drug therapies or treatment modalities for a condition treated on a nursing unit *would* be eligible for CE credit. As a simple rule of thumb, if the activity is required of every nurse on the unit or the department (or even the organization), you probably cannot offer CE credits for the education. (And if you're not sure about CE eligibility, it can't hurt to ask. If you're in a larger organization, you might have a department that can offer CE. If you don't have a department like that in your organization, reach out to your state nurses association, which will have someone on staff who organizes these credits.)

ANCC-APPROVED CONTACT HOURS

Nursing contact hours are awarded by an American Nurses Credentialing Center (ANCC)-approved primary accreditation provider. ANCC-approved contact hours are considered high-quality and evidenced-based educational programs that are free of commercial bias. ANCC accreditation is recognized nationally and internationally as promoting excellence in nursing continuing education. Every board of nursing in the United States requiring continuing nurse education credits for license renewal accepts ANCC-approved credit hours. Regulatory bodies, such as The Joint Commission, and professional nursing organizations requiring CE credit for certification renewal accept ANCC-approved credit hours only.

If you work for an organization that offers at least 15 CE programs per year, you may want to consider seeking approved provider status (contact your state board of nursing to apply). Be sure to weigh the cost of becoming a provider against available educator time, the number of activities/programs offered, and the number of possible learners. Educators who work for organizations that are part of larger healthcare systems should reach out to other educators within the system to plan out the learning activities and educational programs that are needed across the system. What a way to be advocates of standard practice across the continuum of care!

In addition, we suggest checking out free sources of online CE programs specific to your patient population and/or type of nursing that provide approved contact hours for nurses.

As acceptance for Joint Accreditation for Interprofessional Continuing Education grows, completing the application process should become easier for educators because there will be only one process for pharmacy, nursing, and medicine. The Joint Accreditation for Interprofessional Continuing Education is a venture of the Accreditation Council for Continuing Medical Education, the Accreditation Council for Pharmacy Education (ACPE), and the ANCC.

If a learning activity is CE-eligible, offering this credit to learners is a great idea. Offering CE typically increases attendance at the event, and it's tangible evidence of professional development that staff members can place in their professional portfolios. After you decide to offer CE, there are several tasks that require completion before an educational program can be approved for contact hours, beginning with the application.

CE Application

The first step in seeking accreditation is to complete an initial application. Typically, this application is due at least 30 to 60 days before offering the event. To apply for credit hours, staff educators need to demonstrate each of the following:

- The *need* for the CE event, including a gap analysis

- Program outcome

- Method of evaluation

Assessing the Need for a CE Event and Performing a Gap Analysis

A needs assessment demonstrates the need for developing a planned learning activity (check out Chapter 2 for more information on how to perform a needs assessment). In addition to the formal needs assessment, the staff educator should provide literature or evidence that supports the need of providing the learning activity. For example, a needs assessment demonstrates that staff members require an update on new trends in diabetic treatment regimens. Because of many new changes in diabetic care, providing literature or evidence of current trends (American Diabetes Association, *The American Journal of Medicine*, *The Journal for Nurse Practitioners*, *American Journal of Critical Care*, and so on) further demonstrates that nurses are challenged to maintain up-to-date knowledge about best practices in the care of diabetic patients and their families.

As part of the needs assessment, the staff educator must identify the "gap" between the current and desired practice levels by performing a gap analysis. CE approval requires a gap analysis to determine what the education needs are for the program. When doing a gap analysis, the staff educator should ask the following questions:

- What is the overall goal of the educational program?

- What does the audience *need* to know that they do not currently know?

- What does the audience *need* to do that they are not currently doing?

- Is there hospital data indicating an unfavorable trend?

- Are there new treatments or evidenced-based care for chronic conditions?

Using a gap analysis worksheet (see Worksheet 7.1) might assist the staff educator in identifying the gap, as well as the purpose and desired outcome of a learning activity being developed and considered for CE credit hours.

Analysis Step	Description
Desired State	100% of patient education materials will have a 7th grade readability level using Flesch-Kincaid readability tool.
Current State	56% of current patient education materials have a readability level of > 8th grade.
Identified Gap	In 2003, 21% of adults nationally are at a level 1 (< 5th grade reading level). 56% of institution's education materials do not meet the health literacy recommendations (National Center for Educational Statistics).
Gap Due to Knowledge, Skills, or Practice	Lack of knowledge related to health literacy statistics and recommendations. Lack of knowledge on use of Flesch-Kincaid readability tool.
Purpose	Ensure patients and families are provided educational materials that are easy to read and refer to after discharge from hospital.
Outcome Measure	Demonstrate the use of the Flesch-Kincaid readability tool for evaluating patient education materials.

WORKSHEET 7.1   *SAMPLE GAP ANALYSIS WORKSHEET*

Source: Adapted from American Nurses Credentialing Center (2012). Needs assessment and identifying a gap in knowledge, skills, and/or practices. Retrieved from http://cne.nursing.arizona.edu/wp-content/uploads/2014/06/ConductNeedsAssessIdentifyGap-to-resources-online-for-NPs.pptx.

Identifying the Program Outcome

Based on the needs assessment, literature, or other evidence and the gap analysis, the staff educator can develop the program outcome. The *program outcome* is the desired result of the learning opportunity. The program outcome should be measurable and action oriented. Here is an example of an identified program outcome: RNs will identify and understand the use of teach-back to verify understanding of discharge education and apply/incorporate the tool in discharge teaching activities by June 20, 2016.

In addition, the outcome of the activity must be clearly stated and reflect the learning objectives and content of the educational program. For example, a beneficial program outcome might be, "After attending this learning event, participants will be able to apply knowledge and skill in practice related to the diagnosis, treatment, and ongoing management of children with seizures and epilepsy."

To wrap up the CE application process, a summative evaluation is completed and used to assist in planning future continuing education. Many states also require completion of a post-activity report as a means of summarizing attendance numbers, trends in evaluation data, and so on.

Documenting the Method of Evaluation

The type of evaluation will depend on the gap analysis and the content of the learning activity, but in general you would be safe in using Kirkpatrick's Levels of Evaluation (1996), as described in Chapter 6. The following list includes examples of each of the four evaluation levels as they relate to CE applications:

- **Reaction:** This is an evaluation of the general overall satisfaction of a program, or what some refer to as the "happiness factor" of the program. Typically, this evaluation is accomplished by having participants complete a satisfaction questionnaire (could be on paper or online) at the end of the program.

- **Learning:** This is an evaluation of what the learner took away from the program. It's an assessment of new knowledge, skills, or attitudes (KSAs). An example of this type of evaluation is comparing pre- and post-test results or return demonstration (teach-back) of a skill during simulation.

- **Behavior:** This type of evaluation is usually done 6 months or longer after the learning activity. The staff educator assesses for transfer of knowledge into practice. An example of behavior evaluation is to compare pre-test results with post-test results about 6 months after the learning activity or perform direct observation of a skill or an expected behavior 6 months after the learning activity.

- **Results:** This level focuses on the return on investment (ROI). For example, has there been a decrease in errors or costs related to the knowledge or skill presented in the learning activity, or are there improvements in the performance monitors related to the learning activity?

Documenting your evaluation method is part of the CE application process. If for some reason you are unable to evaluate at the chosen level, documentation of the reason you were unable to do so is also important. Keep in mind that forms are not items to make your life miserable, but are actually to be used to demonstrate what is working within your own setting. For example, how often were the activities/ programs evaluated using the behavior level, and how often did using this level demonstrate a positive change in the corresponding results in learner behavior? Trending what works is important!

At this point, your CE application is considered complete, and it's time to submit it for CE credit. Remember, do not leave any of the sections blank or the application will be returned. If you are new to the process, check online to see if the accredited provider you are working with has an FAQ page or email your question to the appropriate source.

CE Development

After the application for CE credit has been accepted, the real work begins. The staff educator now needs to identify learning objectives, develop content, submit disclosures, and create promotional materials for the CE event.

Identifying Learning Objectives

Learning objectives are the expected outcomes the learner will achieve by attending the learning activity. Objectives are measureable and specific as to knowledge gained or skill set achieved by the learner at the conclusion of the program. Each objective should begin with an action-oriented word (for example, demonstrate, apply, recognize, interpret) that relates directly to the program outcome. Generally, there are no more than one or two objectives per hour of continuing education. Some examples of a learning objective would be "Demonstrate the use of the Fry and Flesch-Kincaid readability tools for evaluating patient education materials" or "Explain the methods used to evaluate signs of sepsis in the adult patient."

Developing Content

The learning activity's content should directly correspond with the written learning objectives and should be free of any speaker or company bias. A subject matter expert (SME) should develop the content, which should be supported by evidence. The content should not restate the learning objectives. Instead, the content should provide the information that must be learned in order to meet the stated objective. This information should be listed succinctly in either an outline or a brief paragraph. The best method of delivery is also determined when developing the content. Examples of delivery methods include slide lectures, case scenarios, simulations, role play scenarios, panel discussions, or games/interactive participation.

Submitting Disclosures

In order to ensure the unbiased delivery of educational content to the learners, some safeguards have been put in place to minimize the potential influence of competing interests, known as *conflicts of interest*. Such conflicts can occur if anyone involved in the design, development, or implementation of a learning activity has a financial interest in the content of the activity. For example, let's say you have invited a speaker to discuss the most current pharmacological treatments for diabetes management; however, the speaker is also a pharmaceutical representative for a company that manufactures diabetes medications. In this case, there is a potential conflict of interest, and the presenter would need to disclose this relationship. Planners, speakers, faculty, content experts, and reviewers all need to submit disclosures related to conflict of interest. Disclosures should be submitted well in advance of the learning activity so the staff educator can evaluate the disclosures to determine if there are conflicts and, if conflicts exist, make decisions on how to resolve them. The decision tree shown in Figure 7.1 can assist the staff educator in assessing conflicts of interest.

If a conflict is discovered, resolution of the conflict must occur before the learning activity and awarding of contact hours. The first step is for the staff educator to examine the relevance of the conflict. For example, does a conflict exist when the speaker's name is listed on a speaker's bureau for a medical equipment company but the speaker is providing a learning activity on phone triage skills for transplant patients (where there is no content related to the use of medical equipment)? Because the speaker is not addressing medical equipment or the use of medical equipment, there is no conflict with this learning activity. An example of when a conflict does exist is when a physician is speaking about a specific drug for the treatment of a disease process. This physician is on the advisory board or speaking bureau for the company that produces the medication. In this case, a conflict of interest would exist because the physician may provide biased information during the learning activity.

When a conflict is present, the educator has several options for resolution. The possibilities include not providing contact hours for the speaker's portion of the learning activity, seeking out another speaker, or eliminating from the learning activity any content that is potentially biased.

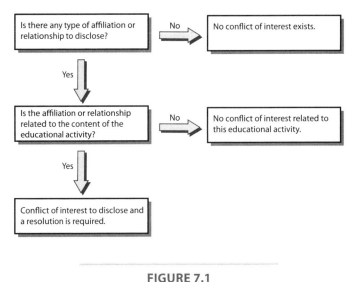

FIGURE 7.1

Conflict of Interest Decision Tree (ONA, 2012).

Creating Promotional Materials

Most continuing nursing education providers approved by the American Nurses Credentialing Center require specific elements in advertisement of approved CE programs (Gorbunoff & Kummeth, 2007). Generally, advertisement of a learning activity offering CE credit hours should include the following key elements:

- Program title

- Speaker

- Date, time, and location of activity

- Program outcome

- Disclosure statement

- Number of contact hours provided

- Accreditation/approval unit number (for example, the Ohio Nurse's Association) and official approved provider statement

- Commercial support (if present)

- Co-providers (if present)

Make sure when creating advertisements for CE-approved educational offerings to refer to the provider's approval manual to include any other specific elements. Thus, how you would market learning activities and educational programs that provide contact hours is different from marketing an inservice, which doesn't require several of the items from the preceding list. That said, you will find it helpful to have a standardized approach to marketing so that something as simple as the time of the event isn't missing from a flyer. If you use the preceding list as a standard, you only need to add whether or not contact hours are being provided to identify the event as an official CE activity.

CE Offering

CE credit hours are calculated on the 60-minute hour. Credit hours only include time that is spent completing the learning activity (content) and evaluating the learning activity. Breaks, meals, and introductions are not included in the calculation of awarded hours. When calculating hours, the planner cannot round up contact hours. For example, if an activity has 3.75 hours of content, the planner can grant only 3.7 content hours (not 3.8 hours). Careful calculation of credit hours should be confirmed with another planner prior to advertisement of the program.

Although this is a general overview of the process to award CE credit hours for learning activities, before applying and advertising an activity associated with accredited CE, you'll want to review any regulations specific to your state or organization to ensure you have met all of the required criteria.

Plagiarism and Copyright Laws

When creating educational materials, the staff educator must always take extreme care not to plagiarize or break copyright laws. *Plagiarism* is "the act of using another person's words or ideas without giving credit to that person" (Merriam-Webster, 2015). Whenever you include others' ideas or words in educational materials, you must clearly acknowledge ownership. Acknowledgment of the source is required even if you're adding a few words, switching the order of words, rearranging sentences, or adapting the material in some other way. Following are some tips to avoid plagiarism:

- Use quotation marks around phrases or sentences that exactly match the original text and provide a citation for the quoted material immediately after the ending quotation mark.

- Paraphrase ideas that belong to others by using your own words. Make sure when doing so you are not copying verbatim more than two or three words of the original work. Again, a citation is required to identify the original source.

- Reference all quotations. For all direct quotations included in your educational materials, provide a complete list of references as the last page(s) of your materials.

As with plagiarism, copyright laws protect works (books, art, pictures, cartoons, graphics, movies or videos, and so on) of authors or creators. If a work is copyright-protected, you must obtain authorization before you can include the work in any educational material. If you're ever in doubt, put in the time and effort to obtain the proper permission before including the material or, if necessary, take the safest route and avoid using the material altogether.

RESOURCES FOR FORMATTING REFERENCES

Here are some of our favorite resources that can assist you in formatting citations and references:

- *Publication Manual of the American Psychological Association (APA, 2009)*

- *Purdue University's Online Writing Lab: https://owl.english.purdue. edu/owl/resource/560/01/*

- *Cornell University's APA Citation Style: https://www.library.cornell. edu/research/citation/apa*

Certification

The importance of certification has increased for the advanced practice nurse. With the APRN role being seen as independent, many state nursing boards require a certification exam as a prerequisite for practice (Chornick, 2008). In addition, because the redesign of health-care includes caring for the patient from cradle to grave, more and more large organizations have facilities across state lines. The concept of having one RN license for all states will rise again. The innovative educator will view certification as being important to the organization on the Magnet journey as well as providing a standard knowledge base for the practicing nurse working within one system across state lines.

We have mentioned in previous chapters that the professional development specialist assists nurses in advancing their knowledge base and careers, but one specific way to help is by promoting certification. The benefits for nurse certification are overwhelmingly advantageous for patients, families, institutions, and nurses. The American Board of Nursing Specialties (2005) mentions that "Certification is the formal recognition of the specialized knowledge, skills, and experience demonstrated by the achievement of standards identified by a nursing specialty to promote optimal health outcomes." Certification gives the nurse credibility in his or her specialty area. Nurses certified in their field of expertise show a higher level of professional development and commitment to their patients. The American Association of Critical-Care Nurses (AACN) points out that while licensure is considered the required first step to providing basic competent nursing care, certification is considered the "expert" step in caring for high acuity patient populations (AACN, 2002). AACN goes on to say that "nurses are ethically and professionally responsible for obtaining specialized knowledge and skills as their careers progress" (AACN, 2002). Consumers are also aware of the value of certification. Consumers seek out hospitals that have a high number of certified nurses. "Americans prefer hospitals that employ nurses with specialty certification. Three in four (73%) said that, given a choice, they are much more likely to select a hospital that employs a high percentage of nurses with specialty certification" (AACN, 2002).

So where does the staff educator fit into promoting certification? The first step is becoming certified in your specialty area (that is, Nursing Professional Development). There is a certification available for nurse educators. The American Nurses Credentialing Center (ANCC) offers certification in Nursing Professional Development. Role modeling the importance of certification to nursing staff makes a strong statement to the importance of certification. It also provides the staff educator with credibility to plan and implement staff development activities. (And for those educators who work at the unit level and provide direct patient care, it might also be wise to obtain certification in that clinical specialty as well.)

The next step in promoting certification to the bedside nurse is by providing information on certifications that are applicable to their practice area. (For a list of nursing certifications, check out http://www.nursingcenter.com/lnc/certification.aspx). For example, if the staff educator works in a critical care unit, he or she would provide information to staff on the critical care certification from the AACN. Raising awareness can occur broadly through flyers or emails, or the staff educator might consider approaching individuals. The latter approach can be a great way to acknowledge an individual's progress, and it sends the learners a message that they are ready to formally demonstrate their achievements.

After promoting interest in certification, the next challenge is to assist staff members in preparing for the certification exam. This will likely require budgetary assistance from the management team. There are many review courses available to help nurses in preparing for a certification exam. There are also review guides and study guides available for purchase (typically available from the certification-offering organization as well as through major bookstores). Many institutions have developed home-grown certification review courses to prepare their staff for testing. Financial assistance or reimbursement for certification is a phenomenal way for an organization to establish the value of certification. The staff educator may need to advocate for reimbursement programs and assist in the development of a reimbursement program.

The final step in promoting certification is providing the certified registered nurse a means of maintaining his or her certification because many certifications require ongoing demonstration of competency for renewal. The staff educator can assist in the development of continuing education (CE) credit activities that meet the requirements of the certification renewal process. The staff educator can also make staff members aware of CE educational programs outside of the organization (for example, at nearby organizations or through conferences and online opportunities).

Professional Nursing Organization Involvement

Many nurses find it difficult to ascertain why they should join professional nursing organizations, and this includes educators. One purpose of these organizations is to determine the knowledge, skills, and attitudes (KSAs) for particular types of nursing practice—critical care, management, infusion nurses, or educators, for example. This in and of itself ties their existence to the subjects of ethics and competency. The ANA Code of Ethics is the overall example for all nurses. To the authors, it means that nurses who are members of professional nursing organizations are leaders because they, by their membership, agree to the standards set by the organization. Members are willing to discuss and reflect on competency for their specific area of practice (Ludwick, 1999), and as we know, nurse competency equals patient outcomes.

Involvement in professional organizations is so beneficial for the staff educator. Professional nursing organizations and associations are "critical for generating the energy, flow of ideas, and proactive work needed to maintain a healthy profession that advocates for the needs of its clients and patients, and the trust of society" (Matthews, 2012). Professional organizations provide nurses with avenues to network and keep up to date with the latest evidence and best practices in their specialty areas. Professional organizations also advocate for nursing issues such as safe staffing, healthy work environments, and standardization of care in specialty areas. There are several professional organizations helpful to the work of the staff educator. Some of our personal favorites include the following:

- **Association for Nursing Professional Development (ANPD).** The mission of ANPD is to "inspire our members to excel by providing educational services, networking, advocacy and research to support the unique needs of nursing professional development" (ANPD, 2015). ANPD provides resources and best practice related to staff development. (See www.anpd.org.)

- **American Nurses Association (ANA).** The ANA's mission statement is "nurses advancing our profession to improve health to all" (ANA, 2015a). The ANA is an organization for all nurses regardless of their specialty area and is dedicated to promoting the highest standards in nursing. (See www.nursingworld.com.)

- **American Association of Critical-Care Nurses (AACN).** AACN's mission is, "Patients and their families rely on nurses at the most vulnerable times of their lives. Acute and critical care nurses rely on AACN for expert knowledge and the influence to fulfill their promise to patients and their families. AACN drives excellence because nothing less is acceptable" (AACN, 2015). AACN sets standards on Healthy Work Environments, providing safe patient care through appropriate staffing and the AACN Synergy Model for Patient Care. (See www.aacn.org.)

- **Sigma Theta Tau International (STTI).** Sigma Theta Tau International's mission is "advancing world health and celebrating nursing excellence in scholarship, leadership, and service" (STTI, 2015). STTI is the first organization to financially support evidenced-based nursing research. The organization continues to support nursing research along with leadership development and education. (See www.nursingsociety.org.)

In addition to your involvement in these organizations, you can also share opportunities with your staff members to join nursing organizations related to the patient population and nursing practice of the unit or department. Why? Because one focus of professional development organizations is to offer current evidence and practice standards in their particular area, thereby assisting their members in maintaining competence through new knowledge specific to the area of practice, awareness of new skills, and even new expectations of the nurse working in a specific type of nursing. For example, the American Academy of Ambulatory Nursing (2014) is guiding the update of its membership to review the Quality and Safety Education for Nurses (QSEN) information and providing links to free modules to complete. In doing so, the organization is agreeing to both the importance of the need for quality and safety in the ambulatory setting and the need for its members to gain new KSAs related to these basic competencies. The staff educator could include the benefits of professional nursing organization membership, such as the following:

- Networking opportunities

- Free or minimally charged continuing education opportunities

- Up-to-date evidence-based or best practice alerts

- Career assistance and opportunities

- Professional development opportunities

- Certification review courses and resources

- Opportunity to attend national conferences at a reduced cost
- Support and mentoring from members of the organization

Leadership and Confidentiality

As a nurse leader, the staff educator provides a safe haven for discussions of concerns and issues that arise on a patient unit. The educator typically does not have disciplinary authority, which is what makes this role safe for a staff nurse when consultation is needed. Because of this, confidentiality is a must. The staff educator must maintain confidentiality related to employee performance issues, performance evaluations, and personal concerns affecting the employee's ability to practice. Just as a direct care nurse would keep confidential that which a patient shares privately, so too does the staff educator respect the wishes of a staff member.

Keep in mind, however, that patient and employee safety always takes precedence over the right to confidentiality (similar to a patient who confides in a nurse that he is thinking of harming himself). A breach in patient or employee safety requires immediate intervention, and, ethically speaking, you would be required to take the issue to the management team for consideration.

Maintaining confidentiality of employee records is another aspect of the educator and learner relationship. An employee's completion (or failed completion) of required education is directly reflected in performance evaluations. Orientation evaluations, test scores, and skills performance reviews are confidential and should not be shared with anyone except the employee and management team. For example, consider a hospital policy that dictates an employee may not work if his or her cardiopulmonary resuscitation (CPR) certification has expired. The employee's failure to complete the CPR requirements by the expiration date is a confidential matter and should not be shared with other staff members.

Record Keeping

Record keeping (or education documentation) can be an overwhelming and time-consuming task for the staff educator. After planning and implementing educational materials, the last thing the staff educator really wants to do is track educational program completions and stay current on other various record keeping. However, having documentation of education completions is a must, especially when accrediting bodies audit your organization. Documents should be readily available during an audit in case evidence of education completion is requested. For example, The Joint Commission (TJC) may be completing an audit involving a patient who was placed in physical restraints. Not only will the surveyor look for appropriate employee documentation in the patient's chart and compliance to the hospital policy regarding restraint usage, but the auditor might also want the staff educator to produce evidence of hospital-required education provided to staff members on the use of restraints and de-escalation techniques.

Every employee should have a paper or electronic education file in which to keep pertinent education materials. Not only should the staff educator have access to the education files but the management team should also have access to these files because most regulatory bodies hold management ultimately responsible for ensuring staff competence. The staff educator should focus on the following areas for record keeping: orientation/initial competency training, regulatory educational requirements, and new equipment training.

Orientation Competency/Initial Competency Training

Orientation records should be maintained in the employee's file for the duration of his or her employment at the institution. Human Resources and Management require that initial employment competencies be on hand for regulatory purposes. This requirement doesn't mean every piece of paper (for example, post-tests) associated with orientation should be kept in the file. A check-off sheet listing required orientation activities, completion dates, and grades, along with employee, educator, and management signatures, is sufficient to document orientation and initial competencies. Unit-specific competencies and practices should also be documented and maintained (especially if the skill has unique unit practice guidelines associated with it).

Regulatory Educational Requirements

Documentation of education mandated by regulatory agencies should be maintained in the employee's file for 3 to 6 years, depending on the regulatory body and organization's human resource policies. Documentation of education includes the course name, date of completion, post-test results (if test included), and any completed skill check associated with the education. TJC and CMS require documentation of education for various topics such as:

- Pain assessment/management
- Restraints
- Blood product administration
- Cultural diversity/considerations
- Patient rights
- Patient abuse and neglect

The educator should work with the organization's department responsible for preparing for regulatory visits to develop a complete list of what education requirements there are for nurses working within that facility. For example, developing a "crosswalk" of those topics required by all regulatory agencies—TJC and CMS, at minimum—would be quite beneficial in mapping out a plan for the upcoming year's education. For those who do not have that luxury, check out the following online resources: TJC's "For Nurses" (http://www.jointcommission.org/nurses.aspx) and CMS (http://www.cms.gov/).

New Equipment Training

New equipment introduced to nursing staff requires competency training and skill assessments related to use of the device and how to perform troubleshooting. When investigating potential device failure or device-related incidents, one of the first items investigated is the nurse's training on the device.

The role of the educator in maintaining competency related to equipment can vary from a simple record maintenance for education to working with the purchasing department and vendor to set up a plan for implementation, and follow-up to evaluate if the equipment is being used appropriately. The educator should have a standardized check-list of what is included in rolling out equipment. This documentation is important in case there is an incident involving equipment and you need to be able to demonstrate the process used for education. Consider including the following:

- Procedure checklist for how to use the equipment (includes where the information is posted for follow-up, including the user's manual)

- List of any of the organization's related policies

- List of areas that will use the equipment

- Percentage of staff required to be educated on the equipment prior to the rollout

- Knowledge that management is aware of the equipment being used in their area, including who has been educated on its use

- Marketing of the education to other professionals who may need to know about its use

- Timeline to adhere to that includes who is responsible for what

Equipment rollouts are a perfect example in which the educator uses project management skills.

Conclusion

Ethic and legal considerations often take a back burner to the educator's daily work. However, in reality, these two items are at the hallmark of what the patient expects, what the organization expects, and what our colleagues expect. The educator who incorporates ethics and legal considerations into education has the opportunity to influence the standardization of nursing behaviors in practice settings. As the academic side of the profession works toward seamless academic progression, and the staff educator works toward growth and development of the clinical practice side, the profession as a whole will be searching for frameworks in which to meet in the middle. Following the ANA Code of Ethics and being aware of legal considerations—whether you are a nursing student, nursing professor, educator, or expert clinician—ensures that professionals adhere to basic principles and the patient receives the care intended.

Questions for Discussion/Reflection

1. In what areas do I role model appropriate ethical behaviors and actions (as per the ANA's Code of Ethics) as a staff educator?

2. How do I as the staff educator keep up on evidence-based practice changes for my clinical area and share/educate staff on these changes?

3. How do I as the staff educator promote a healthy work environment and team building?

4. What staff education have I created that actually could be eligible for CE? What future learning opportunities can I develop for CE credit?

KEY TAKEAWAYS

- *Incorporate ANA's Code of Ethics into learning activities.*
- *Know the process for offering CE credits.*
    - *Promote certification in nursing specialty to role model professional accountability.*
    - *Encourage the benefits of professional nursing organization membership.*
- *Maintain employee confidentiality.*
- *Maintain accurate and complete records with regard to employee education.*

Resources

American Psychological Association. (2009). *Publication manual of the American Psychological Association.* Washington, DC: Author.

Cornell University Library. (2011). *APA citation style.* Retrieved from https://www.library.cornell.edu/research/citation/apa

Paiz, J. M., Elizabeth, A., Wagner, J., Lawrick, E., Moore, K., Anderson, M. … Keck, R. (2013, March 1). *General format.* Retrieved from https://owl.english.purdue.edu/owl/resource/560/01/

References

Accreditation Council for Continuing Medical Education. (2013). Joint accreditation for interprofessional continuing education. Retrieved from http://www.jointaccreditation.org/

American Academy of Ambulatory Nursing. (2014). Enhancing quality and safety nursing competencies in ambulatory care practice. Retrieved from https://www.aaacn.org/enhancing-quality-and-safety-nursing-competencies-ambulatory-care-practice

American Association of Critical-Care Nurses. (2001). Mission and values. Retrieved from http://www.aacn.org/wd/certifications/content/mission-vision.pcms?menu=certification

American Association of Critical-Care Nurses. (2002). Safeguarding the patient and the profession. The value of critical care nurse certification. Retrieved from http://www.aacn.org/wd/certifications/docs/certwhitepaper.pdf

American Association of Critical-Care Nurses. (2015). Nurse certification benefits patients, employers and nurses. Retrieved from http://www.aacn.org/wd/certifications/content/benefitstoptempnrs.pcms?menu=certification#Nurse_Certification_Benefits_Employers

American Board of Nursing Specialties. (2005). A position statement on the value of specialty certification. Retrieved from http://www.nursingcertification.org/pdf/value_certification.pdf

American Nurses Association. (2014). Professional role competence. Retrieved from http://nursingworld.org/MainMenuCategories/Policy-Advocacy/Positions-and-Resolutions/ANAPositionStatements/Position-Statements-Alphabetically/Professional-Role-Competence.html

American Nurses Association. (2015a). About ANA. Retrieved from http://www.nursingworld.org/FunctionalMenuCategories/AboutANA

American Nurses Association. (2015b). Code of ethics for nurses with interpretive statements. Retrieved from http://www.nursingworld.org/MainMenuCategories/EthicsStandards/CodeofEthicsforNurses/Code-of-Ethics-For-Nurses.html

American Nurses Credentialing Center. (2012). Needs assessment and identifying a gap in knowledge, skills and/or practices. Retrieved from http://cne.nursing.arizona.edu/wp-content/uploads/2014/06/ConductNeedsAssessIdentifyGap-to-resources-online-for-NPs.pptx

Association for Nursing Professional Development. (2015). About
ANPD. Retrieved from http://www.anpd.org/?page=about&hhSear
chTerms=%22mission%22

Centers for Medicare and Medicaid Services. (2014). State of operations
manual. Retrieved from http://www.cms.gov/Regulations-and-
Guidance/Guidance/Manuals/downloads/som107ap_a_hospitals.
pdf

Chornick, N. (2008). NCSBN Focus: APRN licensure versus APRN certification: What is the difference? *JONA's Healthcare Law, Ethics,
and Regulation, 10*(4), 90–93. Lippincott Williams & Wilkins, Inc.

Gorbunoff, E., & Kummeth, P. (2007). American Nurses Credentialing Center. (2007). *Nursing professional development review and
resource manual.* Silver Spring, MD: American Nurses Credentialing Center.

Kirkpatrick, D. (1996). Great ideas revisited: Revisiting Kirkpatrick's
four-level model. *Training and Development,* January: 54–59.

Ludwick, R. (1999). Ethical thoughtfulness and nursing competency.
The Online Journal of Issues in Nursing, 5(1). Retrieved from
www.nursingworld.org/MainMenuCategories/ANAMarketplace/
ANAPeriodicals/OJIN/Columns/Ethics/EthicalThoughtfulnessand
NursingCompetency.aspx

Matthews, J. (2012). Role of professional organizations in advocating
for the nursing profession. *OJIN: The Online Journal of Issues in
Nursing, 17*(1), Manuscript 3.

Ohio Nurses Association. (2009). Conflict of interest decision tree. (Infographic). Retrieved from https://www.ohnurses.org/wp-content/
uploads/2014/05/ConflictofInterestDecisionTree_copy.pdf

plagiarism. (2015). In *Merriam-Webster.* Retrieved from http://www.
merriam-webster.com/dictionary/plagiarism

Sigma Theta Tau International Honor Society of Nursing. (2015).
About STTI. Retrieved from http://www.nursingsociety.org/
aboutus/mission/Pages/factsheet.aspx

CHAPTER 8

Putting Technology to Work for You

Introduction

One aspect of the staff educator's role that permeates almost all activities is the use of technology. From personal devices to cloud-based computing and every other level and size of technology in between, what was once the "digital world" is now just "the world." As a nursing professional development specialist, there are many ways you can leverage technology to enhance your role as educator to maximize the learning of your nursing staff. This chapter covers how you might use technology:

- To organize learners' professional development records

- To stay current on the best evidence related to the practice of education, such as the use of technology, specific population cared for in your areas, and changes in nursing practice

- To enhance learning activities

- To meet regulatory agency requirement requests for evidence of individual learner records

Organizing Professional Development Records

Regardless of a professional's role in the workplace, technology can have an enormous positive effect on work-related tasks, helping staff become better organized and more efficient. And technology's impact on the staff educator's day-to-day activities is no less valuable. By using technology to stay organized, educators stand a better chance of doing more *teaching* and less *tracking*, which means educators can make a greater impact on their learners. Although it might be possible to keep learning records on paper if you work in a small office or unit/department with only a handful of employees, this approach has several limitations. Even if you have limited technology capabilities, a simple way to keep your files organized is with spreadsheets. A more robust way to track activities is to use a learning management system (LMS). Both options are discussed in the following sections. You will quickly recognize the importance of record organization when a regulatory organization arrives and requests to view an individual's course records for the past 3 years, or asks to review the list of specific staff who have completed CPR training.

LIMITATION OF PAPER-BASED RECORDS

With the push toward electronic health records in today's U.S. healthcare environment, we think it's safe to recommend you keep at least some level of electronic professional development records. We make this recommendation because paper copies:

- *Are more prone to loss/destruction*
- *Are more likely to contain illegible documentation that could produce erroneous information*
- *Cannot be compiled easily to develop reports for quality or budget measures*
- *Cannot be retrieved easily during an audit*
- *Cannot typically be delivered instantaneously*

Electronic Spreadsheets

Electronic spreadsheets enable users to organize, calculate, and analyze data and then format the results into easily usable information. For staff educators, spreadsheets are useful in tracking learning activities completed throughout the year, as well as tracking nursing license and certification expiration dates, license and certification types, and academic education backgrounds for employees. Using a spreadsheet (such as the one in Figure 8.1) enables the staff educator to easily identify employees' education completions for managers and auditors.

Some staff educators like to post learning activity completion spreadsheets for employees to track and assess their own compliance in educational activities. Educators who want to use this approach must take care to ensure confidentiality, however. Confidentiality can be maintained by assigning each staff member a unique number or other identifier; the staff educator then replaces the employee names on the spreadsheet with the unique identifier. Although this method requires some additional time and effort on the part of the educator, the idea is worth considering. It allows staff members to take accountability for completing required learning activities, and it assists in keeping employees on target by providing a visual reminder.

Although a spreadsheet can certainly be easy to set up and free spreadsheet software is readily available, as the number of staff members you are tracking or the number of learning activities increases, it can be difficult to keep all your records organized. If that becomes the case, you might want to think about using a learning management system.

Learning Management Systems

A *learning management system (LMS)* is commercial-grade software designed to deliver and/or track learning activities for employees. If you are part of a larger organization, you should contact your training/development or human resources department to see if an LMS is available for your use. If one isn't available, it might be worth the cost of purchasing one because it could save the organization quite a bit of money in the long run.

LMSs are made to host a variety of functionality levels. Some of the more basic systems allow only data entry and report generation, but these features are great for producing simple reports (for example, reports needed during an audit by a regulatory agency) or quickly providing employee information when an employee transfers to another department (that employee's new manager would be able to access the employee's record once access was granted).

Cardiac Stepdown FY 2016 Education Tracker

Education/Competency	Restraints 2016	Compliance and Integrity 2016	Cylinder Safety 2016	RN Competency Blitz 2016	Prevention Standards 2016	MRI Safety 2016	Disaster Preparedness 2016	CPR Expiration	CPR Renewal year	Attended Preceptor Workshop	CPN Certification Expiration	Other Certification Expiration	Level of Nursing	School
Alvin	x	x	x	x	x	N/A	x	01/09/17	2017	x	Dec-16		MSN	XU
Angie	x	x	x	x	x	N/A	x	10/31/16	2016		Dec-15		MSN	XU
Anne	x	x	x	x	x	N/A	x	05/10/15	2016	x		Jul-17	MSN	UC
Steve	x	x	x	x	x	N/A	x	03/05/16	2017		Dec-15		MSN	UC

FIGURE 8.1

Sample Learning Activity Completion Spreadsheet

LOOKING FOR A LEARNING MANAGEMENT SYSTEM?

If you don't have an LMS yet, you might want to check out Capterra (www.capterra.com), which provides an overview of many business software applications, including LMSs, as well as reviews. Some healthcare-focused LMSs are provided by Mosby, Lippincott, Angel, and Healthstream.

More advanced LMSs support electronic registration for learning activities, deliver course content within an electronic learning module, allow users to have discussions with each other and content facilitators, or even integrate seamlessly with payroll and performance management documents. Based on the needs and resources of your organization, your facility might even have a few different LMSs, but we would discourage using more than one LMS because one-stop shopping for viewing a learner's activity record can prevent a lot of headaches.

Staying Current

In addition to leveraging technology for organizing employee records, staff educators who want to stay abreast of the most current evidence can use technology to set up a current awareness system. *Current awareness* is a computer science term used by libraries as a means of notifying users (lifelong learners) of newly acquired information, which is often literature. Current awareness is like your own version of an information aggregator that keeps you up to date, and therefore also keeps your learners up to date because you, as the staff educator, are able to incorporate the new evidence *immediately* into orientation, inservicing, continuing education (CE) activities, and so on.

Current awareness is more than good practice. For staff educators who do not have access to free library facilities, it is imperative that they set up a system of current awareness. Why? It is an easy way to stay abreast of topics related to specific patient populations, the practices of education and nursing, and one's specialty, such as ambulatory or acute care. For example, are you aware that the Center to Champion Nursing in America (2010), a collaboration between AARP and the Robert Wood Johnson Foundation, has published the report "Improving Access to Primary Care: The Growing Role of Advanced Practice Registered Nurses," or that the Robert Wood Johnson Foundation

Nursing Research Network (Newhouse, Himmelfarb, Morlock, Frick, Pronovost, & Liang, 2013) supported the report "Improving Rural Hospital Quality by Enhancing Evidence-Based Nursing"? In other words, who do you think has the responsibility for keeping current on information from various sources that should/could affect the practice of education, or the practice of your learners?

Setting up your own system of current awareness (search for "setting up current awareness" online) allows you to subscribe to information, called *feeds*, on topics that *you* want to be sent to you automatically, thus decreasing the time you spend searching for information online. These feeds, also known as *RSS feeds* (real simple syndication feeds), are content listings published by a website. They're used for news and blog websites, but they are also used for distributing other types of digital content, including pictures, audio, or video. Consider setting one up to gather the latest articles on specific topics or have the articles sent to an email address or email folder if you "live" in your email.

There are similar ways to stay updated on new literature through services from the U.S. National Library of Medicine (https://www.nlm.nih.gov). For example, if you have a search strategy where you looked for "pediatric pancreatitis" in PubMed, as new articles become available that meet your search criteria, they can be sent automatically to your email account on a regular basis. One way is to click on the RSS feed symbol located on the top of the page and sign up to receive future articles on pediatric pancreatitis. But first, be sure to conduct a search on "setting up current awareness" and review how to use RSS feeds. The RSS feed symbol looks like a wireless symbol turned on its side.

Another wonderful resource for clinical topics is UpToDate (www.uptodate.com), which contains a large and recent (within the last year) literature review for almost any medical diagnosis. Each review summarizes the information regarding incidence/prevalence, pathophysiology, and treatment and management. Although this service isn't free, if your organization subscribes to it, it's an easy-to-use resource for developing learning activities that include disease-focused information.

Enhancing Learning Activities

The use of technology to enhance learning activities can be challenging when educating multi-generational staff because different generations have a varying degree of comfort levels related to using technology. The Boomer Generation (born between 1945 and 1964) generally have limited use and comfort with technological resources, whereas Net Generation or Millennials (born between 1980 and 2000) have been exposed to technology their entire lives and actually function best when multitasking among devices. As a staff educator, you'll want to think about your learning audience's preferences when considering what type of technology to use in learning activities, as well as how much technology you should use. Although you can't make everybody happy, the use of technology definitely should not *hinder* learning.

In this section we describe and explore a variety of technological tools that you might use with your learning activities so that you are equipped with the knowledge to select the best one(s) that meet your learners' needs:

- Slideshow presentations
- Simulation
- Smartphones
- Tablet (or smartphone) applications
- Social media and video sharing
- Other online resources

Slideshow Presentations

Slideshow presentations using Microsoft's PowerPoint and Apple's Keynote are probably the most common teaching modality used in academic and professional nursing education. Slideshows have come a long way from years past. They can now provide educational content in a variety of ways, such as lectures, gaming, webinar handouts, and asynchronous learning activities (that is, as the basis for developing modules for reviewing in an LMS). If you don't want to pay for products from Microsoft or Apple, you might want to check out OpenOffice.org's Impress, Prezi, and Google's Presentation.

Slideshows enable staff educators to embed technology-based resources such as Internet links, video clips, pictures, and bullet points of information into their lectures. Slideshows provide a means of augmenting the lecture with both auditory and visual cues to assist the learner while still requiring the staff educator to be prepared and knowledgeable about the subject material.

When designing and developing a slideshow, there are several tips to keep in mind. Herrman (2008) recommends the following:

- Use only one typeface throughout the presentation.
- Use at least 24-point font.
- Focus on key words by using animation features.
- For large classes, use a dark background and white or light-colored text.
- Use bullet points rather than complete sentences.

Other general guidelines include the following:

- Include no more than seven lines of text per slide. (More lines require a smaller font and make the slide look too busy.)
- Use no more than seven words per line.
- Stick to sans-serif fonts like Calibri or Helvetica, which are easier to read on a slide.
- Avoid the use of CAPS. Use color to highlight key points instead.
- Avoid underlining words or phrases. Use bold or italics instead.
- Limit animation. Too much creates a busy slide that lacks focus.

Although much of the information in your presentation will likely be text-based, your slides should not be full of words. Graphics, when used to break up text or call attention to a specific piece of information, are an easy way to enhance your presentation. Consider the following guidelines:

- Incorporate charts and tables for describing data results.
- Add illustrations, photos, and other imagery to spice up a presentation. Pictures are great visual cues for learners.
- Embed videos that you recorded using role play or simulation. Videotaped simulations or role play associated with case scenarios can drive home teaching points and promote critical thinking.

- Incorporate or embed clips from YouTube to reinforce key points of the presentation. Remember to consider copyright laws when using YouTube video clips. The website addresses copyright laws and "fair use" of video clips. Works of "commentary, criticism, research, teaching or news reporting might be considered fair use" (https://www.youtube.com/yt/copyright/fair-use.html, current as of March 6, 2015).

FINDING IMAGES THAT HAVE NO COPYRIGHT RESTRICTIONS

If using photos or imagery, make sure you have copyright permission to use items. Remember, just because a photo is on the Internet doesn't mean you can use the photo freely in your presentation. There are several places where you can obtain photos and images that are copyright-free:

- **National Institute of Health.** *Images from this site are public domain, but you must cite the NIH if the image is used. (See https:// imagebank.nih.gov.)*
- **Centers for Disease Control.** *Images from this site are public domain, but you must cite the CDC if the image is used. (See http:// phil.cdc.gov/phil/home.asp.)*
- **MorgueFile.** *Offers multiple free photos that can be used in presentations. (See www.morguefile.com.)*
- **Google Images.** *Search for copyright-free images. (See www. google.com/imghp.)*
- **Yahoo Images:** *Search for copyright-free images. (See http:// images.search.yahoo.com.)*

You can also incorporate clip art provided through Microsoft for PowerPoint presentations or Apple for Keynote presentations, which is generally free to use.

Adding Games to Slideshows

One way for staff educators to make a slideshow more stimulating for learners and to reinforce educational content and evaluate learning is to incorporate gaming. Using gaming as a teaching strategy increases interaction of the learners in a nonthreatening manner—even the quietest learners will speak up. It takes time and planning to set up a game, but there are several ready-to-go, customizable game templates available:

- **Jeopardy.** For example, you could set up an "EKG" round, where answers and questions are related to categories such as Heart Blocks, Atrial Arrythmia, Ventricular Arrythmia, Miscellaneous, and Pacemakers. (See http://www.edtechnetwork.com/ powerpoint.html.)

- **Family Feud.** For example, as part of an interactive orientation, you could set up questions related to organizational policies to help newly hired employees. (See http://powerpointgames. wikispaces.com/PowerPoint+Game+Templates.)

- **Who Wants to Be a Millionaire?** For example, you could use this game as a mini-needs assessment of specific procedures such as blood administration. Since there are specific requirements on how blood is to be administered, playing this game will give the educator information on any knowledge gaps the learners may have. (See http://powerpointgames.wikispaces.com/ PowerPoint+Game+Templates.)

The educator should complete practice runs of the game after it is created to make sure it flows well and meets the learning objectives.

Adding Polling to Slideshows

Embedding polling into slideshows is another method of promoting learner interaction. For example, Poll Everywhere (http://www. polleverywhere.com) uses multiple-choice or open-ended questions to poll and evaluate learners. With this application, the facilitator asks questions, and the learners respond using text to provide instant, anonymous feedback. Based on the answers received, the facilitator can assess current knowledge or evaluate meeting course objectives in real time. The pricing levels for this application are based on the number of participants to be polled and the polling options used.

Simulations

Simulation is defined as "activities that mimic reality of a clinical environment and are designed to demonstrate procedures, decision-making and critical thinking through techniques such as role-playing and the use of devices such as interactive videos or mannequins" (Jefferies, 2005, p. 97). DeYoung (2009) describes the use of scenario-based simulations as a method to assist the novice and experienced nurse in developing or refining critical-thinking skills, improve team communication skills, and provide opportunities to strengthen the ability to complete required skill sets. The staff educator plays many roles in the development of simulations. Oftentimes the educator not only develops the simulation and accompanying scenario used for training but also facilitates the learning activity and conducts the debriefing with the learners after the simulation is completed. Debriefing is the process whereby the learner is provided the opportunity to discuss his/her actions, thoughts, and emotions felt during the simulation. The goal is for the learners to figure out what went well, and what they could have done differently and why.

There are several types of simulators available and they vary widely in cost. Low-fidelity simulation tends to be very skill-focused. An example of low-fidelity simulation is the use of a fake arm to practice intravenous catheter insertion or blood draws. Another example is a mannequin of the head and neck with a tracheostomy to practice tracheostomy care. Simple low-fidelity examples might include using a doll to teach infant or child CPR. Low-fidelity simulation is the least costly type of simulation, but it does require creativity from the staff educator to make the scenario believable.

WHERE CAN I GET A SIMULATOR?

Many companies sell simulators for teaching purposes. Some cheaper options include your local department store where they sell kid's toys and paper plates (some people are surprised at how many dressing changes a paper plate can withstand!). Some more expensive options include companies such as Laerdal (www.laerdal.com), Simulab (www.simulab.com), and CAE Healthcare (www.caehealthcare.com). Many of the simulator manufacturing companies have sales representatives you can contact to get an idea of what level of simulator would meet your needs and how much it would cost.

Moderate-fidelity simulation (MFS) uses a mannequin that has the capability for the learner to listen to an apical pulse and breath sounds. Heart rates, respiratory rates, and breath sounds are usually controlled by a handheld device. MFS does not have eye movement or chest movement. As such, it is often used in competency check-off for basic skills and critical thinking skills. However, if the educator takes the time to create a patient scenario that takes full advantage of the MFS, then this level of mannequin provides the learners with the opportunity to increase their ability to care for specific patients. For example, staff often struggle with recognizing the signs and symptoms of sepsis. Yet by the time sepsis is diagnosed and the patient is transferred to the ICU, it is very often too late. In such a case the educator could write a scenario that includes the importance of noting a change in vital signs over a short period of time, and the learner is able to practice steps to take when there is a change using the MFS.

High-fidelity mannequins are the most expensive simulators, but they provide the most realistic learning opportunity. High-fidelity mannequins are computer-based and typically require multiple resources to manage. Not only do you need a facilitator to run the simulation scenario but generally you also need an operator to run the simulator. Using a computer, the operator can make the mannequin speak to the learner and then adjust vital signs in response to interventions performed. High-fidelity mannequins also aid in improving assessment skills. The learner will have the ability to auscultate heart and breath sounds, see the chest rise and fall, and feel palpable pulses. The mannequins are quite realistic and can be used for high-level simulations. However, high-fidelity simulators require space, maintenance, and additional manpower resources when conducting the actual simulation.

There are several advantages and disadvantages to the use of simulation for learning activities. The number-one advantage is the ability to practice skills and team communication through scenario-based simulation in a safe environment. No harm to a patient occurs, and learners actually feel they are in a "real" situation and can act accordingly. Learners have the ability to problem solve and apply concepts of previously learned knowledge into the simulation. The major disadvantage is cost, not only for the cost of the simulator but also costs related to their use, which include classroom or storage room costs, training on use of the simulators, maintenance fees, and manpower to complete the simulation. Another disadvantage is that simulators can provoke anxiety and intimidate some learners, especially the baby boomer generation of learners.

The Planning Process

Using simulation as a teaching strategy requires a lot of pre-planning. Campbell and Daley (2013) recommend that the key elements in Worksheet 8.1 be used as a guide in creating a simulation. The goal is to create a simulation to be as "real" as possible.

To see how these considerations can produce a full learning activity with simulation, check out one of our examples in Table 8.1.

Guiding Questions	Additional Considerations
What is the title?	Title of the simulation. Include a brief description of the course.
What is the focus of the simulation?	Assess competence of a skill? Communication and team building? Evaluation of new equipment or new process? Performance evaluation? Test out of a class? Development of critical-thinking skills?
What is the scenario description?	What are the patient demographics? Sex/age/gender/race? Height/weight? Allergies? Past medical history? Past surgical history? Past psychological history? Medications? Social history/significant others? Reason for patient encounter or admission?
What are the scenario objectives?	Team-building objectives; critical-thinking objectives; skill or performance objectives.
What will I need to set up the scene?	What type of simulator (adult/child/infant; low-, moderate-, or high-fidelity)? How many staff members will I need to run the simulation? What roles will be played in the simulation (RN, MD, Charge RN, Respiratory Therapist, etc.)? What equipment will I need to run the scenario? What paperwork will I need for the scenario?
What is the scenario to be implemented?	Create the following pathways: (a) Expected pathway—successful outcome, (b) Alternative pathway—took extra steps to have a successful outcome, (c) Alternative pathway—took wrong steps with unsuccessful/poor outcome.
What are the evaluation criteria?	Were objectives met? Debrief participants, including such things as: Overall feelings of the scenario? What went well? How did the team function? What could have gone differently? What alternative decisions could have been made within the team? Did the team have all of the resources necessary? Were there process issues that can be addressed? How did the communication among the team feel? Did everyone on the team have the same mental model? What are individual team members' takeaways?

WORKSHEET 8.1   *CREATING SIMULATION SCENARIOS*

TABLE 8.1 EXAMPLE OF SIMULATION PREPARATION

SCENARIO COMPONENT	DETAILS SPECIFIC TO THE SCENARIO
Goals and objectives and technical and nontechnical	Recognizes SVT rhythm and initiates PALS treatment protocol…vagal maneuvers, notifying cardiology resident team, preparing for Adenosine administration
	Recognizes decompensation/changes in perfusion assessment
	Recognizes need for synchronized cardioversion
Target participants (roles, specialty)	RN, PCA, HUC and cardiology residents, fellows, and attendees
Clinical setting	Patient room-in-situ
Basic scenario information (outline)	Seven-week-old infant admitted from clinic with 1 week history of ↑WOB, poor feeding tolerance, and fussiness. Found in clinic with HR of 220 bpm, which terminated in clinic without intervention. SVT documented by EKG in clinic. Patient admitted to unit for continued monitoring and management of SVT. Infant's weight is 3.5 kg.
Simulator to be used	Infant
Fluids and medications	Saline well with flushes
	Adenosine ordered for bedside
Equipment needed (IVs, ET tubes, chest tubes)	Saline flushes 1 ml syringes Stop-cocks Defibrillator Oxygen/infant NC Mapleson bag with infant mask Code sheet DASH monitor with pulse ox

SCENARIO COMPONENT	DETAILS SPECIFIC TO THE SCENARIO
Paperwork, labs, X-rays, EKGs, photos, videos	EKG-SVT
Medication intervention	Adenosine: 0.1 mg/kg and then progress to second dose of 0.2mg/kg Normal saline flushes/bolus
Airway intervention (oxygen, BVM, intubation)	Mapleson bag/infant mask…to bag if necessary Infant NC while in rhythm
Physiologic intervention (CPR)	
Procedures and other interventions	Cardioversion with 0.5–1 J/kg, if ineffective, ↑ to 2 J/kg
Number of and education of instructors	
Evaluation tools and measurement points	
Advance organizer/pretest and how delivered	
Personnel-simulation specialist, actors/family members	
Estimated time to run simulation and debriefing	20 minutes
Need for re-evaluation (time frame)	Debrief for approximately 20 minutes

Figure 8.2 provides an example of evaluation criteria for the educator to use during a specific simulation. It is important for the educator to determine how the scenario will be implemented, evaluated, and reinforced in practice. Education should be applied as soon as possible in the practice setting once completed, or at the end of a set timeframe. For example, when education is delivered to the entire organization, a timeframe for completing the simulations is set. Doing so helps reinforce the new learning and makes all staff educators (as colleagues) ask questions of each other once they know others have completed the simulation experience. Thus, criteria such as that listed in Figure 8.1 is constantly reinforced both in the simulation and practice settings.

ASSESSING EQUIPMENT NEEDS FOR A SIMULATION

The medical equipment needed to carry out a simulation varies by scenario. What follows is a generic list of equipment that might be required for a simulation:

- *Patient monitor*
- *Equipment to assess vital signs (blood-pressure cuff, stethoscope, pulse ox probe, monitor leads)*
- *Oxygen (O2) and associated O2 equipment (cannula, non-rebreather, ambu bag)*
- *Suction setup and suction catheters*
- *Medications for expected use*
- *Intravenous (IV) lines and fluids*
- *IV pumps, syringe pumps, feeding pumps and drain bags (collection reservoir) for the IV fluids used during scenario*
- *Other tubes or drains (intubated endotracheal [ET] tubes or tracheotomy tubes, chest tubes, indwelling urinary catheters, Jackson-Patt drains [JP drains])*
- *Traction setup*
- *Dressing supplies*
- *Emergency/crash cart*

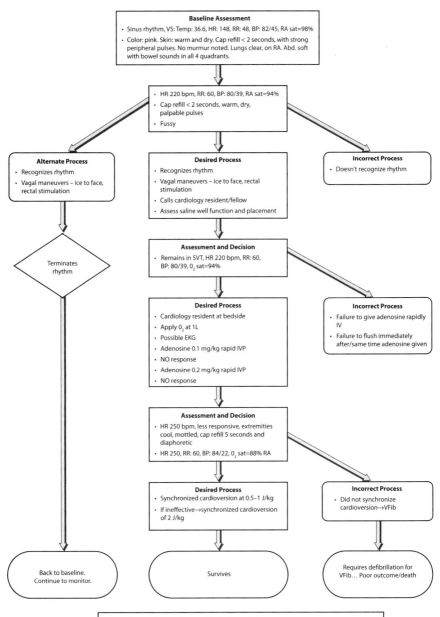

Baseline Assessment
- Sinus rhythm, VS: Temp: 36.6, HR: 148, RR: 48, BP: 82/45, RA sat=98%
- Color: pink. Skin: warm and dry. Cap refill < 2 seconds, with strong peripheral pulses. No murmur noted. Lungs clear, on RA. Abd. soft with bowel sounds in all 4 quadrants.

- HR 220 bpm, RR: 60, BP: 80/39, RA sat=94%
- Cap refill < 2 seconds, warm, dry, palpable pulses
- Fussy

Alternate Process
- Recognizes rhythm
- Vagal maneuvers – ice to face, rectal stimulation

Desired Process
- Recognizes rhythm
- Vagal maneuvers – ice to face, rectal stimulation
- Calls cardiology resident/fellow
- Assess saline well function and placement

Incorrect Process
- Doesn't recognize rhythm

Terminates rhythm

Assessment and Decision
- Remains in SVT, HR 220 bpm, RR: 60, BP: 80/39, O_2 sat=94%

Desired Process
- Cardiology resident at bedside
- Apply O_2 at 1L
- Possible EKG
- Adenosine 0.1 mg/kg rapid IVP
- NO response
- Adenosine 0.2 mg/kg rapid IVP
- NO response

Incorrect Process
- Failure to give adenosine rapidly IV
- Failure to flush immediately after/same time adenosine given

Assessment and Decision
- HR 250 bpm, less responsive, extremities cool, mottled, cap refill 5 seconds and diaphoretic
- HR 250, RR: 60, BP: 84/22, O_2 sat=88% RA

Desired Process
- Synchronized cardioversion at 0.5–1 J/kg
- If ineffective→synchronized cardioversion of 2 J/kg

Incorrect Process
- Did not synchronize cardioversion→VFib

Back to baseline. Continue to monitor.

Survives

Requires defibrillation for VFib... Poor outcome/death

- Vital signs and interventions associated with each step should be delineated.
- Additional steps and processes may be added; this is an example.
- Evaluation points and fatal flaws should be annotated.
- Process may transition from one line to another (incorrect to desirable or vice versa).
- Time frames prior to transition from one step to another should be delineated along the arrows.

FIGURE 8.2

Example of Simulation Flow/Progression

The Debriefing Process

Debriefing in many cases is considered the most important aspect of simulation. It is a time to reflect on the learners' experiences and provide constructive feedback. Debriefing allows the participants to analyze the events in a safe environment that unfolded during the scenario. It also allows an opportunity to ask clarifying questions related to the scenario. Because simulation is supposed to be very similar to real-life situations, debriefing allows the participants to express emotions felt during the scenario and provides a "cool-down."

The following list includes some discussion questions that facilitate debriefing:

- Was Medical Response Team (MRT) or Rapid Response Team (RRT) code called?

- Did you know who the team leader was, and as the team leader, how did you feel?

- How did the team function? What were the team's strengths? Weaknesses?

- Discuss how well the team communicated. Did everyone on the team have the same mental model?

- Was there closed loop communication/repeat back of orders? Give examples.

- What were some of the challenges? Why?

- Did you have all the resources needed for this scenario?

- What are the team members' takeaways?

Debriefing is most effective if done immediately after the simulation has been conducted. When done immediately after the simulation, the scenario, emotions, and actions taken are fresh on the participants' minds. Discussion and reflection, therefore, is much more meaningful. Debriefing should take about 20–30 minutes and should be incorporated in the planning of the simulation timeline. This length allows time for the participants to discuss their feelings and takeaways.

A Safe Learning Environment

Another consideration when running simulations is the importance of creating a safe learning environment. Some staff members might feel that if they act inappropriately or inaccurately in front of a manager, there will be repercussions related to their performance. Therefore, unless the simulation is being used to evaluate performance, members of management or leadership teams should not be included in the learning activity. Eliminating management participation makes the environment safer and the learner less anxious of the learning activity. The facilitator should have a discussion prior to the simulation that explains "what happens in the room, stays in the room." Some organizations have staff sign confidentiality forms to drive home the point of a safe learning environment.

Smartphones, Tablets, and Apps

The use of smartphones in patient care areas is beginning to replace the use of pagers and other communication devices. Smartphones can be used not only as a source of communication among team members through voice and texting capabilities but also as a means of communicating changes in patient-monitoring parameters. Some organizations have started using smartphone technology and smartphone applications to relay patient-monitor alarms and even go as far as displaying patient waveforms on the smartphone's screen.

Smartphones can also be used to assist the staff educator in training, providing resources for staff members, and evaluating learners' knowledge or application of concepts. The staff educator needs to play an active role in determining how the phones can be used to reinforce what is taught in orientation, inservicing and continuing education activities. For example, imagine there is a change to the organization's policy on caring for the patient with an indwelling urinary (Foley) catheter. To help with implementation of the new policy, the staff educator could potentially send a text message with three questions to charge nurses who can review and discuss the messages at shift report with oncoming staff members.

Other emerging technological opportunities come to the staff educator in the form of apps used on tablets such as the iPad (Apple), Surface (Microsoft), Galaxy Tab (Samsung), or the Kindle Fire (Amazon). According to online MobiHealthNews' report "Q4/2013 Year-End State of the Industry Digital Health" (2014), there are 5,820 medical, health, and fitness apps available for smartphones today. Staff educators will want to work closely with their information technology staff to stay abreast of what is approved for use by the organization, as well as educating nurses to ask patients what apps they are using and why.

There are many apps that are available as a resource for nursing staff or to use in association with other educational modalities by the staff educator. An example of a useful app is Heart Murmur Pro, which helps nurses learn how to auscultate heart murmurs. The app provides pictures of where murmurs are best heard, best location for stethoscope placement, and audio sounds of the murmur. The learner can compare normal heart sounds to the murmur for differentiation. This app could be used in conjunction with a case scenario during a lecture, small group just-in-time learning, or one-to-one review with a staff member. A few other cardiac apps available include PALS Review, PALS Advisor, PALS Mobile Assessment Wizard, ACLS Advisor, ACLS Megacode, Critical Care ACLS Guide, 3M Littmann SoundBuilder, and ECG Pocket Reference.

Tablets also have a wealth of resource applications. These apps provide the staff educator and nursing staff with resources at their fingertips using either tablets or smartphone technology. Some of the more useful apps available for resources that we really like include:

- **Medscape.** Provides reference tools for diseases and conditions, procedures, and drugs, as well as medical news and continuing medical education courses.

- **Centers for Disease Control and Prevention (CDC) Mobile activities.** Provides up-to-date information such as important health articles, Disease of the Week, prevention tips, and updates timed with important health concerns.

- **PICU Doctor.** Serves as an app version for the PICU Cardiac Guide and contains information about topics such as physiology, ventricular assist, or anesthesia as they relate to pediatric intensive care.

- **Medical Dictionary.** There are several medical dictionary apps to choose from; some require purchase. The overall goal of these apps is to improve your knowledge about medical terms and concepts.

- **MicroMedex.** Serves as a resource for drug interaction compatibility, including IV. There are several versions; some require purchase.

- **Gray's Anatomy.** Serves as an anatomy textbook resource. Again, there are several to choose from, including a student version; some require purchase.

- **Nursing Reference Center.** Serves as a reference for evidence-based information.

- **Lexi-Comp.** Serves as a resource for drug information such as IV compatibility and drug interactions. May require purchase.

For any app that requires purchase, check with your librarians to learn if the app was included in a purchase of another reference. In addition, you might consider adding iMedicalApps to your current awareness to stay abreast of the latest reviews of new medical apps.

Social Media and Video Sharing

Although social media should never be used to communicate with or about individual patients, it can be used as a means of notifying nurse learners about upcoming learning activities. For example, Facebook can be used to create educational events and outline the curriculum for learners to register or access online, and Twitter can be used to make brief announcements and create excitement around an activity. In addition, many schools of nursing and large organizations have their own YouTube channels with member-only access. Nursing procedures can be video recorded and accessed as a reference for bedside staff members. Patient education videos can also be created and shared with patients and families as part of self-care and discharge education. Staff educators working in smaller organizations might want to see what's available on YouTube or Google Video for access to free content that provides instruction on many nursing procedures.

Additional Online Resources

The Web provides a wealth of free online resources that staff educators can use to support the content of their work. Here are a few of our favorites:

- **QR codes.** Placed on equipment, these codes can link to your policy/procedure manual and provide learners with a simple how-to checklist or specific safety information.

- **Infographics.** Short for "informational graphics," these elements provide a visual representation of information or important facts about a topic of interest. For example, an infographic could include information about student athletes and head trauma. They frequently appear in poster format, so you can post them in break rooms, patient rooms, and so on.

- **SlideShare.** SlideShare is a website that staff educators (and other professionals) can use to both post and retrieve content such as slideshow presentations or research projects. Part of the educator's professional development is to share with and learn from others—just be sure to give proper credit for what you use. (See www.slideshare.net.)

- **PowToon.** This software allows you to create animated cartoons that can be inserted into a slideshow presentation, posted to a video sharing site, or even your organization's website. (See www.powtoon.com.)

- **Screen Cast-o-Matic.** A free online resource, this software enables you to audio record over your slideshow presentations, and it acts as a host for your presentations. (See www.screencast-o-matic.com.)

- **Edmodo.** This free online resource provides a way to organize your learners and help them stay connected to you. (See www.edmodo.com.)

Staff educators who work in smaller organizations or rural settings or who don't control their own budgets might benefit from exploring and investigating these free online resources. We have seen firsthand how these resources help staff educators organize their work. Consider picking one or two to pilot.

Caring for Patients

When technology in nursing became more than heart/respiratory monitors, the nursing profession's concern was forgetting about the patient. Articles about "high tech, high touch" were written in the 1980s, and they continue today. There is an art and science to nursing. The use of technology assists the science of nursing, giving nurses all kinds of information that allows them to provide the art of caring to the patient. To the educator this means that they must incorporate components of caring, such as how and when to communicate, into learning tasks. For example, when writing simulation scenarios, shouldn't the educator include phrases to help calm the patient? There is nothing more calming to a patient in any healthcare setting than another human's touch. In today's environment we are all about texting for communication and the use of technology to "see" how the patient is faring. The educator who is able to combine technology and touch will succeed in developing a caregiver responsible and accountable for desired patient outcomes.

Electronic Medical Records

Proper documentation is critical to the care of the patients and is one of the interprofessional competencies for all healthcare disciplines. Although the currently available electronic medical records (EMRs) often do not meet the needs of the healthcare workers or the patients on a daily basis, they do often provide data for the staff educator to use as both a means of education assessment and content application evaluation.

You might consider working with other organizational leaders to determine when a change in the EHR should be added to initial orientation. Stakeholders responsible for programs and projects all believe their own projects are the most important and should be taught to all new employees. It is helpful to have ranking criteria and a method to guide you in these decisions. We have provided an algorithm to help with this decision-making in Figure 8.3.

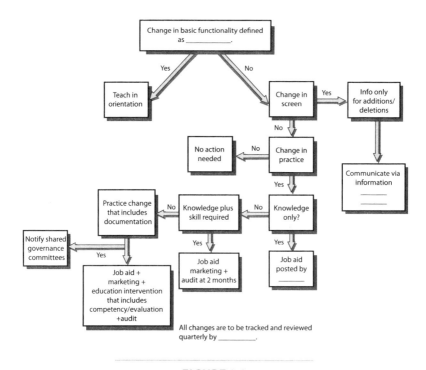

FIGURE 8.3

Decision Tree for Determining When to Include EMR Changes in Orientation

New Equipment

Just as the technologies for communication, teaching/learning, and documentation continue to change, so, too, do the technologies used in equipment for patient care. As new equipment becomes available, there are several considerations for which a staff educator is responsible. Most of these follow the use of the ADDIE model for teaching something new as well as unique documentation requirements (which were mentioned in Chapter 7).

However, keeping up with these technology changes (and even staying ahead of them) is beneficial for the staff educator. We recommend getting to know your equipment sales representatives very well so that they know to contact you whenever your organization is considering the purchase of new equipment. Also, when you attend national conferences, check out the exhibits for the latest and greatest in patient care equipment so that you know what's out there and what might be coming to your organization soon. Finally, consider being a part of the equipment selection team at your organization (or become friends with a manager or staff educator who is already part of that team). Staying knowledgeable about equipment considerations will give you ample time to become familiar with the technology before being required to help staff members learn how to operate it.

Conclusion

Technology has really broadened the horizons in staff development and nursing education. Nurse educators can now track education electronically by using spreadsheets or by using learning management systems. Nurse educators can enhance what used to strictly be lectures to using interactive slideshows. Technology now enables staff educators to use a simulated setting to practice skills, improve communication, encourage team building, and promote critical thinking. This can all be done in a safe environment with no harm to patients. One of the most useful aspects of technology is that resources are now at our fingertips through the use of smartphones and tablets.

Questions for Discussion/Reflection

1. How can I track employee education more easily with the use of technology?

2. How can I incorporate simulation into unit-based education?

   - In orientation?

   - For developing critical thinking?

   - For developing team building?

   - For promoting critical-thinking skills?

3. How can I use technology to make my slideshow presentations meet multiple learning styles?

KEY TAKEAWAYS

- *The educator needs to understand when to use the different types of technology in developing and designing education, as well as understand what technology the learners will need to know to adopt the new education into their practice.*

- *The educator needs to begin with the end in mind in determining which technology to use to create the education. What domains of learning will be the focus? Is there only a cognitive component? Or a psychomotor skill plus an affective component?*

- *The educator needs to ensure that the use of simulation includes evaluation that begins with debriefing and continues in the clinical setting by reinforcing how the simulation learnings support the current nursing practice as well as the growth and development of the individual learner.*

References

Campbell, S. H., & Daley, K. (2009). *Simulation scenarios for nurse educators: Making it real.* New York, NY: Springer.

Center to Champion Nursing in America. (2010). Improving access to primary care: The growing role of advanced practice registered nurses. Washington, DC: Author. Retrieved from http://campaignforaction.org/sites/default/files/2010.FS_.ImprovingAccesstoPrimaryCareAPRNs.pdf

DeYoung, S. (2009). *Teaching strategies for nurse educators.* Upper Saddle River, NJ: Prentice Hall.

Herrman, J. (2008). *Creative teaching strategies for the nurse educator.* Philadelphia, PA: F. A. Davis Company.

Jefferies, P. (2005). A framework for designing, implementing, and evaluating simulations used as teaching strategies in nursing. *Nursing Education Perspectives, 26*(2), 96–103.

MobiHealthNewsResearch. (2014). Q4/2013 Year-end state of the industry digital health. (2014). Retrieved from http://mobihealthnews.com/research/quarterly-reports/state-of-the-industry-digital-health-q4year-end-2013/

Newhouse, R., Himmelfarb, C. D., Morlock, L., Frick, K. D., Pronovost, P., & Liang, Y. (2013). *Improving rural hospital quality by
enhancing evidence-based nursing.* Princeton, NJ: Robert Wood
Johnson Foundation. Nursing Research Network. Retrieved from
http://www.rwjf.org/en/library/research/2013/08/improving-rural-
hospital-quality-by-enhancing-evidence-based-nur.html

YouTube. (n.d.). What is fair use? Retrieved from https://www.youtube.
com/yt/copyright/fair-use.html

INDEX